The Bigger They Are, The Harder They Fall

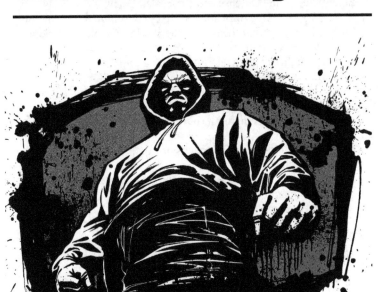

How to Fight a Bigger and Stronger Opponent in the Street

Sammy Franco

Also by Sammy Franco

Self-Defense Tips and Tricks
Kubotan Power: Quick & Simple Steps to Mastering the Kubotan Keychain
The Complete Body Opponent Bag Book
Heavy Bag Training: Boxing, Mixed Martial Arts & Self-Defense
Gun Safety: For Home Defense and Concealed Carry
Out of the Cage: A Guide to Beating a Mixed Martial Artist on the Street
Warrior Wisdom: Inspiring Ideas from the World's Greatest Warriors
Judge, Jury and Executioner
Savage Street Fighting: Tactical Savagery as a Last Resort
Feral Fighting: Level 2 Widow Maker
The Widow Maker Program
War Craft: Street Fighting Tactics of the War Machine
War Machine: How to Transform Yourself Into a Vicious and Deadly Street Fighter
First Strike: End a Fight in Ten Seconds or Less!
1001 Street Fighting Secrets
When Seconds Count: Self-Defense for the Real World
Killer Instinct: Unarmed Combat for Street Survival
Street Lethal: Unarmed Urban Combat

The Bigger They Are, The Harder They Fall
Copyright © 2014 by Sammy Franco
ISBN: 978-0-9853472-0-8
Printed in the United States of America

Published by Contemporary Fighting Arts, LLC.
P.O. Box 84028
Gaithersburg, Maryland 20883 USA
Phone: (301) 279-2244
Visit us Online at: www.SammyFranco.com

For author interviews or publicity information, please send inquiries in care of the publisher.

Contents

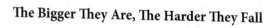

"However big the whale may be, the tiny harpoon can rob him of life."

- Malaysian proverb

Warning!

The information and techniques in this book can be dangerous and could lead to serious injury. The author, publisher, and distributors of this book disclaim any liability from loss, injury, or damage, personal or otherwise, resulting from the information and procedures in this book. This book is for academic study only.

Preface

The Bigger They Are, The Harder They Fall is a comprehensive text that confronts the daunting task of fighting a larger and stronger adversary in a street fight. As you thumb through these pages, you will quickly notice that this book was written for the serious self-defense practitioner who wants to develop the skills and expertise necessary to effectively trounce a massive and menacing adversary.

It's ironic that with the hundreds of martial art and self-defense books that flood our bookstores, nothing has ever been specifically written about this crucial aspect of self-defense. Nevertheless, if you are serious about "real world" self-defense, you need to read and study this book.

This book is divided into five chapters. Chapter One addresses the basic concerns of fighting a larger and stronger opponent. Topics include the three factors of combat victory, the folly of steroid use, controlling panic and intimidation, the masking technique, developing confidence, combat attributes, somatotypical advantages and disadvantages, and proficiency forecasts.

Chapter Two provides you with the strategic principles necessary to do the job right. Topics include: striking power, weapons of choice, offensive considerations, first strike and the compound attack, the necessary mind-set for fighting a massive enemy, targets and reaction dynamics, distance of combat, mobility and footwork, defensive considerations, and putting it all together.

Chapter Three tackles the arduous task of training you for the big fight. Here, I will address warming up procedures, over training and burn-out, training partners, mental visualization, cardiovascular training, weight training, workout routines, equipment training, the three training methodologies, and specialized sparring drills.

Chapter Four shows you the strategic principles put into action. Here, you will see, step by step, how to take him down and out of the fight! In this chapter, I have provided 12 street-fighting scenarios demonstrating the appropriate techniques and methods of destroying a redoubtable adversary.

Chapter Five covers the inevitable ground fight. Here, I address the many critical issues surrounding grappling and ground fighting a larger and more powerful adversary. Topics include: ground-fighting risks, defending against a charging assailant, countering the body tackle, escaping from the leg guard and mounted positions, nuclear ground-fighting tactics, positional asphyxia, and escaping from standing grabs and chokes.

Bear in mind that the terminology in this book is defined within the context of Contemporary Fighting Arts and its related constituents. Therefore, I have included a detailed glossary at the end of the book. Please refer to it as needed.

Unlike other self-defense textbooks, The Bigger They Are, The Harder They Fall is easy to follow and understand. For reasons of simplicity, I have taken the liberty of writing this book in a question and answer format. When used accordingly, it will provide you with the technical know-how to cope and ultimately defeat a hulking adversary. Since this text is both a skill-building workbook and strategic blueprint for combat, I firmly encourage you to make notes in the margins and underline passages.

Finally, I strongly recommend that you read this book from front to back, chapter by chapter. Only after you have finished the entire text should you treat it as a reference and skip around, reading those chapters that interest you.

- Sammy Franco

The Bigger They Are, The Harder They Fall

Chapter One
Important Questions

"The most formidable weapon against errors of every kind is reason."

-Thomas Paine

You are probably very eager to get down to some serious training. But wait! Before you begin your program, you need to read this chapter. Here I will address the fundamental concerns of fighting a larger and stronger adversary in a street fight. Besides answering some critical questions, it also serves as a psychological primer that will prepare you for the upcoming chapters.

Q: Is it really possible for a smaller or weaker person to defeat a larger and stronger person in a street fight?

A: Absolutely. While size and strength are critical factors in a street fight, they are not the only determining factors. There are many other variables that play a material role in determining who will win.

Q: Exactly which factors determine who wins a self-defense altercation?

A: There are three factors that play a major role in who wins a violent self-defense confrontation. They are knowledge, skills, and attitude. Knowledge means knowing and understanding how to fight. Skills refers to psycho motor proficiency with the various tools and techniques of combat. Attitude means being emotionally, philosophically, and spiritually liberated from societal or religious mores that would prevent you from injuring, maiming, or killing your adversary.

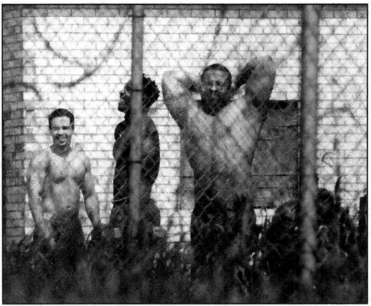

Our prison system breeds large and powerful criminals. In this photograph, Riker's Island inmates worked out. (Photo by wide world photos.)

Q: You refer to the words "street fight." Is this the same as a self-defense situation?

A: A street fight, by definition, is a spontaneous and hostile confrontation between two or more individuals where no rules apply. It is a sudden, violent encounter that can occur anywhere and at anytime. Therefore, "street fight" and "self-defense situation" should be treated as one in the same.

Q: Do I have to be a skilled martial artist to defeat a larger and stronger opponent in a fight?

A: No. If you are reasonably intelligent, possess a modicum of athletic ability, and study the principles in this book, you will do just fine. Actually, they are some martial artists who are more likely to be injured or killed because they rely on impractical and ineffective techniques. In many ways, the average layperson is much better off than he is.

Q: What about using an equalizer? Why don't I just use a knife or gun against him?

A: Every self-defense situation is going to be different and no two street fights will ever be the same. There are just too many variable and factors that must be taken into consideration when deciding how much "force" to use in a self-defense confrontation. As a matter of fact, many self-defense situations do not justify the use of deadly weapons such as knives or guns.

Keep in mind, *just because your adversary is larger or stronger than you, doesn't legally or morally justify the use of deadly force.* Unfortunately, this is a truth and a reality that you must come to terms with. So, if you want to avoid going to jail and doing time in prison, you better be very careful when handling and using deadly weapons.

Q: What about using less lethal weapons like pepper spray, stun guns or a kubotan mini stick?

A: There's no doubt these self-defense weapons can be very effective under certain conditions. However, you must not fall victim to dependency - the sole reliance on a particular self-defense weapon for personal protection. Remember, all self-defense weapons have limitations and they will most likely not be with your when you need it most. The truth is, your mind and boy are you best self-defense weapons.

Q: What about using mixed martial arts (mma) techniques against a larger or stronger opponent?

A: Unfortunately, mixed martial arts (both professional and recreational) are geared exclusively for sport competition. They are not designed for dangers of real-world self-defense. As a matter of fact, mixed martial arts have "technique restrictions" and students and practitioners must follow specific rules and regulations. Actually, there's a very good reason why there are specific weight divisions in mixed martial arts competition.

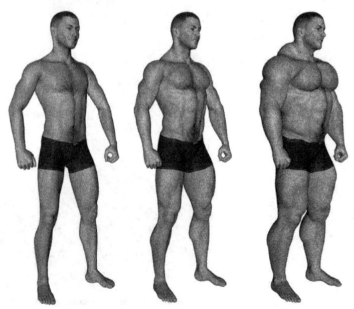

When it comes to mixed martial arts, bodyweight and size play a critical role in the outcome of a match. Would a Welterweight (left) mixed martial artist really want to fight the man on the right?

As I discussed in my book, *Out of the Cage: How to Beat a Mixed Martial Artist on the Street,* body weight, body size and somatotype play critical roles in the overall effectiveness of many MMA techniques. If a mixed martial artist was forced to fight a behemoth in the streets, he would quickly realize that many of his grappling and ground fighting techniques would be ineffective against his larger foe.

Q: What if my opponent uses steroids and is exceptionally strong?

A: First, it is important to understand exactly what steroids are. Essentially, anabolic steroids are synthetic chemical compounds that resemble the male sex hormone testosterone. When incorporated with a high-intensity weight-training program, this "performance-enhancing" drug is known to increase lean muscle mass, strength, and endurance in most men. Most anabolic steroids are taken in pill form; however, some are taken by injection. Many users will cycle steroids (taking the drugs for six to 12 weeks then stopping for a period of time before starting again). While steroids might give your adversary freakish size and/or strength, you can still defeat him if you employ the information found within this book.

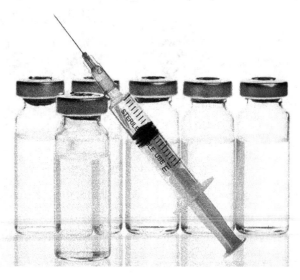

The Bigger They Are, The Harder They Fall

Q: If steroids give my opponent such a great advantage, should I consider taking them?

A: Only if you have a death wish! Anabolic steroids produce terrible side effects and even short-term use of such drugs can be extremely harmful, even fatal. Here are some possible side effects: liver damage or cancer; high blood pressure; reduction of HDL, the "good" cholesterol; gastrointestinal disorders; headaches and nosebleeds; gagging and vomiting; jaundice; baldness; gynecomastia (over development of the breast tissue in males); impotence; acne; bad breath; increased chance of tendon, ligament, and muscle injury; violent and homicidal mood swings known as "roid rages"; severe depression; and muscle cramps and spasms.

Q: Is it normal to panic when faced with a monstrous adversary who wants to kick my ass?

A: Yes and no. If you are unprepared and faced with an overwhelming adversary, it is normal to experience mild panic. You will most likely question your abilities, and you may feel frustrated, apprehensive, and intimidated. But, I can help you with this.

Q: How can I avoid being intimidated by a bigger guy?

A: Intimidation is generally caused by a lack of confidence. And confidence can only be acquired through preparedness. Preparedness is the only thing that will give you an unshakable belief in yourself and your abilities to defeat your adversary. There are three components of preparedness that must be mastered—cognitive preparedness, psycho motor preparedness, and affective preparedness.

Cognitive preparedness requires you to be mentally equipped with the strategic concepts, principles, and general knowledge of combat. I will address cognitive preparedness in great length in Chapter Three.

Psychomotor preparedness requires you to be physically prepared for the rigors of close-quarters fighting. It means possessing all the physical skills and attributes necessary to fight and defeat a stronger adversary. There are many exercises and drills that will help you achieve psycho motor preparedness, and they are discussed in Chapter Two.

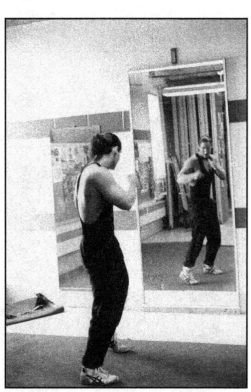

Psychomotor preparedness requires you to be physically prepared for the rigors of close-quarters fighting.

Finally, affective preparedness requires you to be emotionally and spiritually prepared for the strain of combat. It means philosophically resolving issues related to combat so your attitudes, ethics, and values harmoniously orchestrate with the paradoxical task of fighting. Now is the time to sit down and find

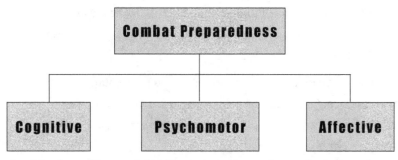

Acquiring the confidence to fight a bigger opponent can only come from preparedness. Here are the three essential components of preparedness that you must possess.

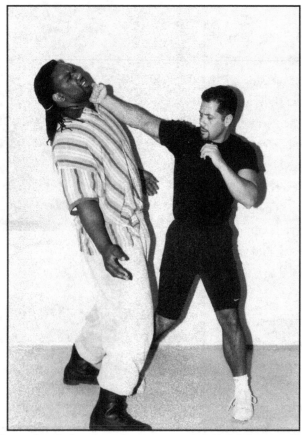

Preparedness is the only thing that will give you an unshakable belief in yourself and your abilities to defeat your adversary. In this photo, the author delivers a lead hook to his attacker head.

clear and lucid answers to questions concerning the use of violence in self-defense.

Keep in mind that by closely following the tactics and principles in this book, you will acquire the three components of preparedness and be immune to intimidation.

Q: What if I can't help being intimidated? Is there anything else I can do?

A: Yes - try masking. Masking is the process of concealing your true feelings or emotions during the pre-contact stage of fighting (in this particular case it would be fear or panic) from

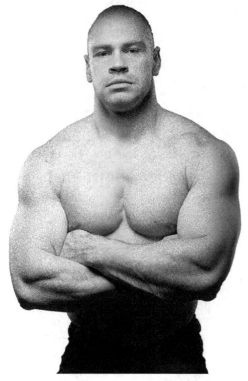

There is no doubt that a larger and stronger man has a big advantage in a street fight. Despite what you may have heard, size does matter.

your opponent by manipulating and managing your body language (both facial and body expressions).

Masking is a learned skill that requires your constant attention. When faced with a massive adversary, you cannot afford to have a momentary lapse in your body language. You must be aware of yourself at all times. You must appear strong and confident, regardless of the fear you are experiencing at the moment.

The Bigger They Are, The Harder They Fall

While masking cannot cover or hide all involuntary physical reactions (such as excessive perspiring, heavy breathing, and trembling hands and legs), you can cover them up by quickly moving about or diverting the assailant's attention elsewhere.

Q: I read somewhere that self-confidence goes a long way in self-defense. Is this true?

A: It's true, so long as it's *legitimate* confidence. You must believe in your ability to fight and always convey a strong sense of confidence to your enemy. Confidence is critical in every facet of combat because it permits you to fight in the face of extreme adversity. Despite the odds and circumstances, you have to be optimistic about your ability to neutralize your adversary.

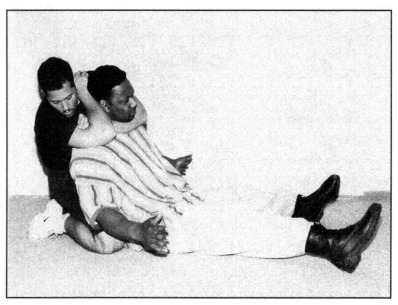

Anyone can be taken out in the street fight, regardless of how big or strong he may be. If you possess the knowledge, skills and attitude, you can defeat a massive adversary in a self-defense situation. In this photo, the author applies a rear choke hold on his adversary.

Preparedness, accompanied with a high degree of self-esteem, will help you avoid entertaining thoughts of self-doubt or apprehension. Negative self-talk is the greatest saboteur of self-confidence; listening to these negative internal messages during a street fight will hinder your ability to fight. Make every effort to prevent these messages from entering your mind.

Q: I have often heard some well-known fighters and teachers say, "There's always someone out there who can beat you." Do you agree?

A: I don't think it's a question of agreeing or disagreeing. I think it really has to do with your perspective and outlook. For example, if you subscribe to this philosophy of defeatism, there's a very good chance you will make it come to fruition. I'm sure you've heard of the term "self fulfilling prophecy." However, this is not to say that you should live in denial or have a warped perspective of your self-defense skills and abilities. Nevertheless, my philosophy and approach is to always go into a fight with the absolute certainty that you will win and come home alive.

Q: From a psychological and strategic point of view, what do I need to defeat a larger opponent?

A: You'll need proper planning, intelligence, raw courage, and the focused aggression of the killer instinct.

Q: From a physical point of view, what is necessary for defeating a larger opponent?

A: Combative attributes play a big role. Combative attributes are the various mental and physical qualities that enhance your combat skills. Some attributes include strategic development, physical conditioning, range proficiency, striking power, target orientation, and explosiveness (more will be discussed in the next chapter).

Q: What advantages do larger and stronger men have in a street fight?

A: Since a larger man carries more body weight, he will have significant power in his strikes and blows. He will also most likely have a reach advantage, allowing him to strike you from a greater distance. If he has some appreciable height, his facial targets may be difficult to reach and strike. Moreover, a larger man's body can

LARGER AND STRONGER MAN

Advantages when fighting

- Greater striking power
- Greater appendage reach
- Limited facial targets
- Better grappling ability
- Significant ground fighting advantage
- Pre-contact psychological advantage
- Body can withstand greater punishment

Disadvantages when fighting

- Generally slower appendages
- Weaker stability when standing
- Greater torso & leg target exposure
- Greater telegraphic potential
- Often cocky & overconfident
- Limited "in fighting" ability
- Slower mobility and footwork skills
- Actions are less court defensible

generally absorb more punishment than a smaller man's.

The skeletal and muscular structure of a massive adversary is an important consideration. Because of his size and weight, his bones are going to be larger and stronger; the cortexes of these bones are going to be substantially thicker and will be able to withstand greater punishment. The thick, powerful neck muscles weld his head to his shoulders, enabling him to withstand significant impact to the head and face region. Body fat is another significant factor. If you are fighting an overly fat opponent, remember that his body fat will act as a shield that protects his muscles and nerves from the force and impact of your blows. In addition, because of his large mass and extra body weight, he will have several advantages in a ground fight regardless of his skill level. More will be discussed in Chapter Three.

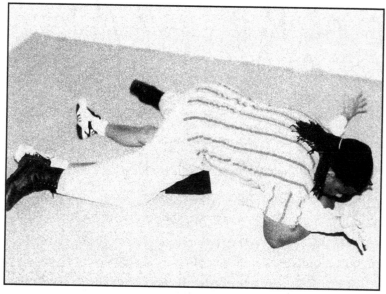

Beware! A larger opponent can easily smother you during a ground fight. Be especially careful when fighting in this range of unarmed combat.

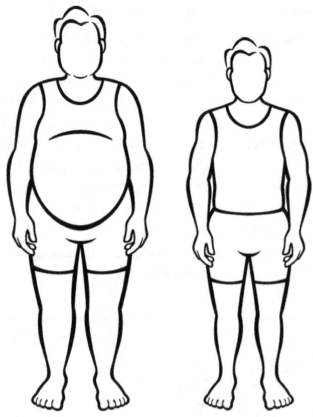

If you are fighting an overly fat opponent, remember that his body fat will act as a shield that protects his muscles and nerves from the force and impact of your blows. Which one of these two men has the advantage of withstanding body blows?

Q: Does a larger man have any disadvantages?

A: In most cases, a larger man's movements will tend to be a bit slower than his smaller counterpart. For example, if he were to throw a kick, it would take longer to initiate because his limbs are longer and must move a greater distance to be chambered. Since a taller man's center of gravity is further away from his support base, he has a greater chance of compromising his stability in his stance. A tall man's legs and torso can also be particularly vulnerable to attack. Finally, a larger man usually has a false sense of security by placing too much emphasis on his brawn and not enough on skill and strategy. He often makes the mistake of underestimating smaller opponents.

Q: Are there any advantages for a smaller person when fighting a bigger guy?

A: Since a smaller man will have shorter appendages, his arm and leg movements will generally be quicker and less telegraphic. His footwork will usually be more rapid than his larger counterpart. Since he is smaller, he has less target exposure than his hulking counterpart.

SMALLER OR WEAKER MAN

Advantages when fighting

- Quicker appendage movement
- Less telegraphic potential
- Rapid footwork and mobility
- Minimal target exposure
- Greater stability and balance
- Better (striking) in fighting ability
- Greater chance of witness intervention
- Greater court defensibility

Disadvantages when fighting

- Limited appendage reach
- Generally poor confidence
- Easily intimidated
- Limited long-range fighting ability
- Limited ground fighting arsenal
- Weaker standing grappling strength
- Body can't withstand punishment

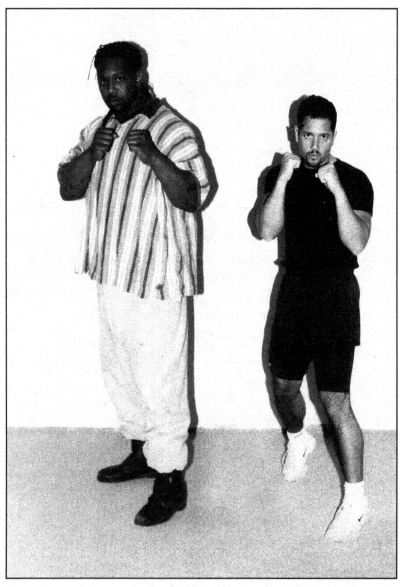

There is less target exposure for a smaller fighter. Do you see any differences between the two men in this photograph?

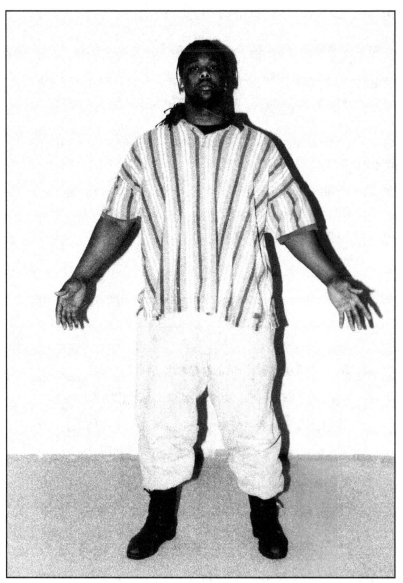

A massive opponent has the very same anatomical targets that you and I have. The eyes, nose, chin, throat, groin, and knees are just a few.

The Bigger They Are, The Harder They Fall

His legs and torso are not as vulnerable to attack. Because a shorter man's center of gravity is closer to his support base, he is more likely to maintain stability in his stance. Finally, if your opponent decides to take you to court and sue you for damages, a jury is more likely to look favorably on a smaller man than a larger one.

Q: What are the disadvantages of being the smaller person in a street fight?

A: The smaller person tends to become intimidated when confronted by a larger and stronger man. As a result, his fighting ability and performance drops significantly. Unless the smaller man is well trained in ground fighting, his larger adversary will have the advantage in this range of combat. Last but not least, a smaller man will not have the reach advantage of his larger counterpart.

> **In the streets, confidence goes a long way! Remember, your opponent is less inclined to pick a fight with you when you radiate a confident (not cocky) demeanor. Giving off bad vibes like fear and trepidation and apprehension will only strengthen your opponents resolved to hurt you.**

Q: Are there any examples of smaller people defeating larger adversaries?

A: Sure. The annals of history are of full of examples. David vs. Goliath, Jack Dempsey vs. Jess Willard, Max Baer vs. Primo Carnera, Rocky Marciano vs. Joe Lewis, and Mike Tyson vs. Larry Holmes.

However, the best example I can give you, is the simple fact that women are threatened and attacked by larger and stronger men on a daily basis. As you might expect, the ones who are properly trained are the ones who come home alive.

Q: Since we're on the subject, what is the best type of physique for reality based self-defense?

A: Before I can answer this question, you must understand the somatotypes of combat. Basically, the human body is categorized into one of three different physical body types known as somatotypes: the ectomorph, the mesomorph, and the endomorph.

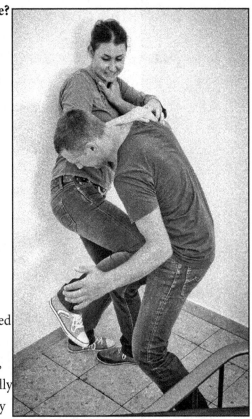

Ectomorph: Characterized by elongated arms and legs, narrow chest and shoulders, thin, long muscles, and generally low body fat. He is usually the weakest of the three body types.

Being threatened and attacked by a larger and stronger person is more common than you think. In fact, women deal with it on a regular basis.

Mesomorph: Characterized by a large chest and torso, appreciable musculature, and considerable strength. He is generally the strongest of the somatotypes.

Endomorph: Characterized by a "soft" appearance, round face, wide hips, and a considerable amount of body fat.

Keep in mind that some people can be a combination of all three somatotypes. For example, a well-muscled football player who carries some body fat would be classified as an endo-mesomorph. In reference to the above question, the ideal type of body for unarmed combat would be a pure mesomorph.

Q: How long will it take me to learn the skills to beat a bigger guy?

A: There is no clear-cut answer to this question since the time it takes to become proficient varies according your own skills and abilities. However, by following the principles and strategies outlined in this book, you will accelerate the learning process dramatically. Let's move to Chapter Two and get started.

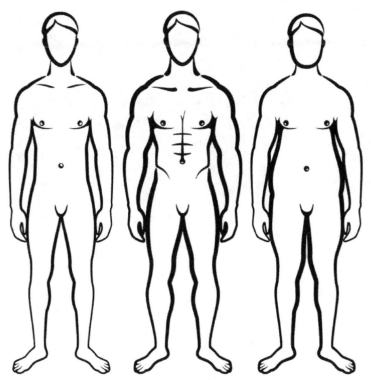

The human body is categorized into one of three different physical body types known as somatotypes. From left to right: the ectomorph, the mesomorph, and the endomorph.

The Bigger They Are, The Harder They Fall

Chapter Two
The Game Plan

"It is a bad plan that admits of no modification."

- Publilius Syrus (1st century B.C.)

Now that we have addressed the basic questions of fighting a larger and stronger opponent, it is time to move on to the specific strategy and tactics of beating him.

In this chapter, I will equip you with the strategic principles necessary to confront and ultimately defeat a massive opponent in a street fight. It is designed to give you the confidence and clarity of mind necessary to take immediate control of the fight and end it quickly and decisively. As soon as you grasp these fighting concepts, you'll be able to launch forward with a practical and effective method of attack.

Let's begin by discussing the necessity of striking power.

Striking Power is Vital

Q: What is the most important physical attribute when fighting a larger adversary?

A: There are actually many important attributes for hand to hand combat. However, the first one that comes to mind is striking power. If you have nothing behind your strikes and blows, you will be in serious trouble. It's vitally important for you to have the necessary power to stop your opponent from continuing his aggressive actions.

Just like a home defense firearm, you must possess the "stopping power" necessary to immediately neutralize an intruder. The very same concept applies to self-defense in the streets; you cannot afford to have weak or otherwise ineffective self-defense techniques that don't get the job done.

Q: Can a smaller person generate as much striking power as a bigger person?

A: Yes indeed! Striking power is not predicated on just size and strength. You don't have to be a heavyweight prize fighter or some oversized football player to have power.

While it's true that body weight can substantially increase your striking power, it's not the only determining factor. For example, take a look at the late Bruce Lee (five foot seven and weighed approximately 130 pounds) who could hit harder than most heavyweight boxers. Lee was able to do this because of two important factors. First, he mastered the fundamentals of body mechanics and technique. Second, Mr. Lee exploited the laws of kinetic energy by relying on movement speed instead of body weight to generate his

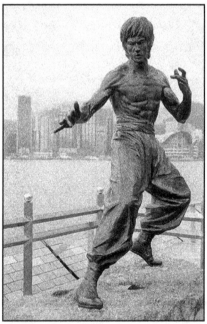

There's no doubt that Bruce Lee knew a thing or two about striking power.

impact power.

Bruce Lee's freakish explosive power can actually be validated by understanding the basics of kinetic energy. Essentially, mass (m) times (v) velocity equals impact power. If you double the mass of the object (i.e., body weight) and leave the velocity (speed of the punch) constant, you will double the impact power. But, if you leave the mass of the object (i.e., body weight) constant and double the velocity (speed of the punch) you will quadruple the power.

Mass x Velocity = Impact Power

Q: Is there anything else I can do to maximize the power of my punches?

A: Yes. There are several other principles that will further enhance your striking power. In fact, by learning proper fighting technique and understanding how to employ your three power generators, you can actually punch harder than a larger man!

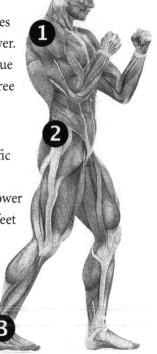

Essentially, power generators are specific anatomical points that will maximize your body torque. There are three anatomical power generators: the shoulder (1), hips (2), and feet (3). By properly synchronizing these three body parts, you will significantly increase both the force and penetration of your blow.

Another effective method of increasing your punching power is to step forward as you deliver your blow (i.e., lead straight, rear cross, palm-heel strikes, etc.). Remember, however, that this technique will only work if your punch is executed simultaneously as you step toward your adversary. This will take some practice and training but with time it can become second nature.

Q: Any more tips?

A: Sure, I can give you a few more. First, your punch or strike must be accurately delivered to its target. Second, it must be delivered rapidly, without any hesitation. Third, you need to properly time your blow so it is delivered at the precise correct moment. Fourth, you must keep your muscles relaxed while delivering your offensive technique and only during impact should you tense your fist (remember to relax, then contract). Fifth, exhale as you deliver your strikes. Sixth, you must remember to "snap" your blow into the selected target. Finally, you must hit with your entire body (using your three power generators), not just your arm.

Q: What is the best piece of training equipment for developing punching power?

A: The heavy bag is unsurpassed for developing powerful striking techniques. (For more information, see Chapter Three.)

Q: What about those "dim-mak" strikes that can kill a man instantly? Are they worth looking into?

A: Those supposed "death touch" strikes do not exist. I repeat, **do not exist!** They are one of the many ridiculous martial art myths that have been floating around for decades. You have to remember, the human body is a very powerful and resilient structure. It does not just drop to the floor by the touch of a hand. It is simply impossible. As I have said, the only effective and efficient way to incapacitate a powerful adversary (when you are employing punching techniques) is to shower him repeatedly with bone-shattering blows directed toward vulnerable target sites.

Techniques You Need to Know!

Q: Do I need a lot of different fighting techniques to beat a larger and stronger opponent?

A: No. There are only a few techniques that you need to master. Actually, the fewer techniques you need to know, the better. When it comes to self-defense training, always keep it simple.

Q: Which punches or strikes are particularly effective against a larger adversary?

A: There are five that I recommend. They are the finger jab, web-hand strike, hook punch, shovel hook, and uppercut. Let's take a look at each one.

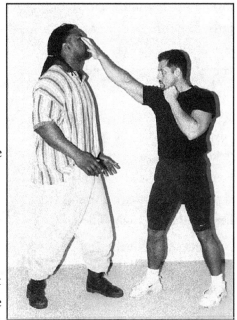

Finger jab strike: A quick, non telegraphic strike executed from your lead arm. Contact is made with your fingertips. To execute the finger jab properly, quickly shoot your arm out and back and remember not to tense your muscles before delivering the strike. The target for the finger jab is

The finger jab is a versatile self-defense technique that can be deployed in both punching and grappling ranges of unarmed combat.

the assailant's eyes. Regardless of the opponent's size and strength, the finger jab can cause temporary or permanent blindness, severe pain, and shock.

Web-hand strike: A devastating technique that can be delivered in both punching and grappling ranges. Depending on the amount of force, a strike to the opponent's throat can cause gagging, excruciating pain, loss of breath, nausea, and possibly death. To deliver the strike, simultaneously separate your thumb from your index finger and quickly drive the web of your rear hand into the adversary's throat. Be certain to keep your hand stiff with your palm down. Once contact is made, quickly retract your hand to the starting position.

The Hook Punch: One of the most devastating blows in your arsenal. To execute the hook punch, quickly and smoothly raise your elbow up while simultaneously

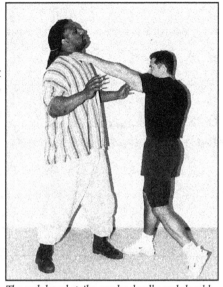

The web hand strike can be deadly and should only be used in life and death self-defense situations!

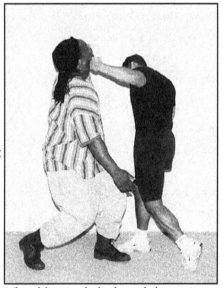

When delivering the hook punch, be certain your arm is bent at 90° and that your wrist and forearm are kept straight throughout the execution of the movement.

torquing your shoulder, hip, and foot into the direction of the blow. As you throw the punch, be certain that your fist is positioned vertically. Also, remember to follow through your target. Depending on the target that you hit, the hook punch can cause severe pain, loss of breath, nausea, unconsciousness, concussion, shock, coma, and possibly death.

The Shovel Hook: This punch travels diagonally into your assailant's face or torso. To properly execute the shovel hook, dip your shoulder and simultaneously twist your leg and hip into your assailant's target, then drive your entire body into the assailant. Again, keep balanced and follow through your selected target. Once again, depending on the target that you select, the hook punch can cause severe pain, loss of breath, nausea, unconsciousness, concussion, shock, coma, and possibly death.

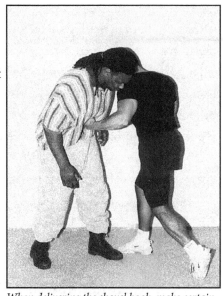

When delivering the shovel book, make certain to put your body into the below and follow through your selected target.

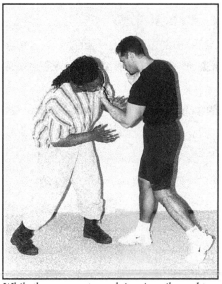

While the upper cut punch is primarily used to "chop the opponent down" by attacking his torso, it can also be used for head strikes.

29

The Uppercut: Another severe blow, the uppercut can be delivered in both punching and grappling ranges. This "fractal tool" travels in a vertical direction to either the assailant's chin or body, and it can be delivered from both the lead and rear arm. To execute the uppercut, quickly twist and lift your body into the direction of the blow. Make certain the punch has a short arc and that you avoid chambering your blow. When delivered properly, the uppercut should feel like an explosive jolt. A properly delivered uppercut can cause severe pain, loss of breath, concussion, shock, and unconsciousness.

LESS IS BETTER!

When it comes to unarmed self-defense, less is always better. The self-defense techniques that you use in a street fight must be simple and usable under the stress of real-world combat conditions.

Q: Why are these five self-defense techniques so important?

A: The finger jab and web-hand strikes are superlative because they are efficient and non telegraphic first-strike tools that can be delivered to the opponent's upper targets.

The hook punch, shovel hook, and uppercut blows are also excellent tools for attacking the opponent's torso targets. These three circular strikes generate centrifugal impact force that can knock your opponent out cold with only a minimal amount of effort.

Q: Should I use open-hand strikes or fisted blows when fighting?

A: You will need to use both to get the job done. Open-hand strikes (finger jabs, web-hand strikes, palm heels, etc.) are primarily used as first-strike tools, while fisted blows (lead straight, rear cross, hook punches, etc.) will comprise your secondary strike arsenal. I discuss this important distinction in my book, *First Strike: End a fight in Ten Seconds or Less!*

Q: I recently attended a reality-based self-defense seminar where the instructor told us not to throw fisted blows in a fight. He said punching techniques are risky and will cause a severe hand injury when fighting.

A: To the uninitiated this may sound logical and prudent observation, but in reality it's a big mistake that will drastically hinder your ability to effectively protect yourself or a loved one from harm.

In real world self defense, you need to be able to hit your opponent, from a diversification of angles, vantages, and distances of combat. The only way to accomplish this essential requirement is to possess an arsenal of fisted blows that can shower the opponent from all possible angles.

There's good reason why mixed martial arts fighters and boxers rely heavily on punching skills and techniques. When executed

BEWARE!

Beware of the martial arts or self-defense instructor who tells you that open hand strikes alone are sufficient for self-defense. This person has obviously never experienced real combat.

correctly, punching is a highly efficient form of fighting.

The bottom line is, if you want to be able to protect yourself from a larger and stronger adversary, you must master the science of punching.

Q: So, is it true that I can injure my hands when punching?

First, you must understand that any time you decide to fight back against an attacker, you always run the risk of injury. It's just the price of doing business in the streets.

Essentially, there are four main causes of punching related hand injuries. They are weak structural integrity of the fists, poor skeletal alignment of the hands, wrists and forearms, and

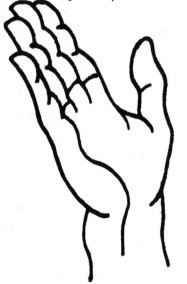

Open hand strikes, like palm heels, are safer to deliver than most fisted blows however, neutralizing an opponent of superior size and strength will require both open and assisted self-defense techniques. There is no other way around it!

hitting the wrong anatomical target. While there are different body mechanics for each and every punch, there are four things that must take place in order to avoid a hand injury. They include the following:

- Knowing how to make a proper fist.

- Strong hands, wrists and forearms.

- Maintaining skeletal alignment when your fist makes contact with its target.

- Hitting the proper anatomical target and avoiding contact with extremely hard boney surfaces.

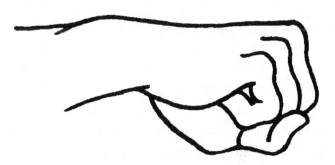

When using fisted blows in a fight, be certain to keep your hand and wrist aligned with your forearm. If your wrist bends on impact, you could seriously injure it.

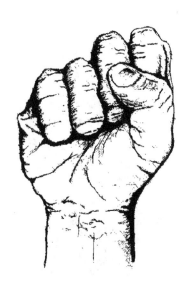

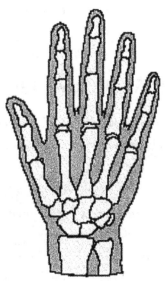

This is a classic mistake made by beginners. Notice how the index and middle finger protrude from the fist. When making a fist, make certain that all of your fingers are clenched evenly. Your knuckles should be flat like a brick.

The human hand is not as strong as you might think. One assisted below makes contact with the opponent's skull, it can easily result in a hand fracture. Therefore, it's essential that all assisted blows are delivered accurately and at the right moment.

Q: Is there anything else I can do to reduce the chances of bending or spraining my wrists when throwing punches?

A: Strengthening your wrists, hands, and fingers can help. Not only will strong wrists and hands improve the structural integrity of your punch, but strong fingers will also improve your tearing, crushing, and gouging techniques. Moreover, strong hands will improve both your weapon retention and disarming skills. One of the best methods of strengthening your wrists and hands is to regularly squeeze a tennis ball; 200 repetitions per hand would be a good start.

Q: What about choking techniques? Can I use them against a bigger opponent?

A: As a matter of fact, you can. The rear naked choke, for example, is an excellent technique that can be used against an opponent of any size. For more information, see chapter five.

Offensive Considerations

Q: Can I use your self-defense techniques with a mixed martial arts or boxing stance?

A: Actually, you can. The offense techniques that I mentioned earlier can be used with just about any stance. However, if you want to maximize your chances of winning and minimize your chances of losing, be certain to use a practical fighting stance. Avoid using flowery or exotic martial arts stances that expose your centerline.

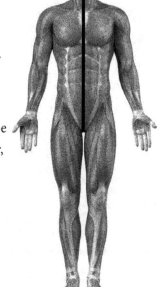

The centerline

Q: Can you recommend a good fighting stance?

A: Sure. Actually, I teach a variety of different stances or postures. In this case, I'll teach you a basic fighting stance used for unarmed self-defense. This fighting stance is important for combat because it is a strategic posture that facilitates maximum execution of your body weapons while simultaneously protecting your targets against possible counter strikes. In unarmed street fighting, the fighting stance is used for both offensive and defensive purposes. It stresses strategic soundness and simplicity over complexity and style.

The fighting stance is very easy to put into practice. To assume the stance, position your feet and body at a 45-degree angle to the adversary. If you are right-handed, keep the right side of your body facing your adversary. Next, place both your feet approximately shoulder width apart with both knees bent and flexible. Keep both of your hands up and align your lead hand in front of the rear hand. Stay relaxed and loose and remember to keep your chin angled down. And don't forget to keep 50% of your body weight distributed evenly over each leg.

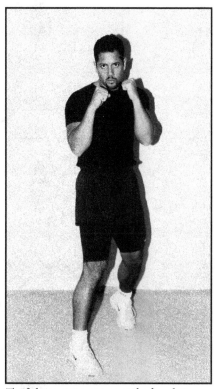

The fighting stance serves as the foundation of your striking arsenal. Here, Sammy Franco demonstrates the proper hand and foot positioning.

35

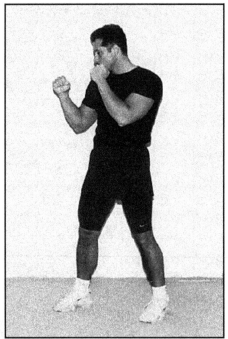

Pictured here, a side view of the fighting stance.

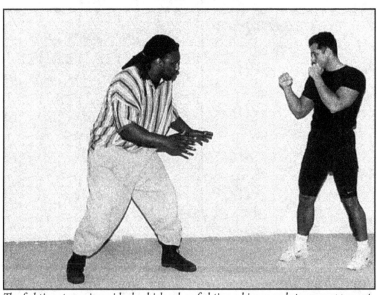

The fighting stance is an ideal vehicle when fighting a bigger and stronger opponent. In this photo, the author squares off with his 300 pound adversary.

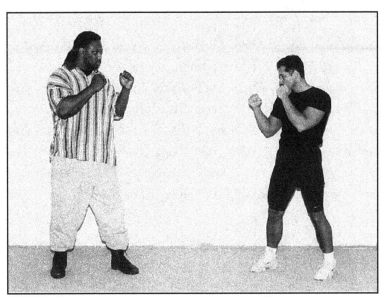

With the popularity of mixed martial arts, there's a very good chance your opponent will know how to square off in a fighting stance.

THE IDEAL FIGHTING STANCE SHOULD:

- **Provide stability**
- **Provide mobility**
- **Provide balance and motion**
- **Facilitate rapid deployment of offensive and defensive techniques**
- **Offers a noncommittal weight distribution**
- **Doesn't unnecessarily tax your muscles**
- **Looks intimidating to the adversary**
- **Feels relatively comfortable to the practitioner**

The Bigger They Are, The Harder They Fall

Q: I once heard that there is no such thing as a perfect fighting stance for street combat. Is this true?

A: Yes and no. There is such a thing as a "perfect" fighting stance in training because you have the time to adjust and articulate your body in accordance with the standards of proper form. There is no pressure or threat of real danger at the moment. However, in real life combat where things are fast and uncertain, there is no such thing as a perfect stance. When all is said and done, you take what you can get under the circumstances of your fighting situation.

Also, keep in mind, there might be circumstances that prevent you from assuming a protective stance. For example, if you are caught off guard by a surprise attack. In such a situation, you don't have time to "set up" a fighting structure. Instead, you would have to react immediately without any foundational reference point. This is one of the reasons why I teach my students to defend themselves both with and without a stance.

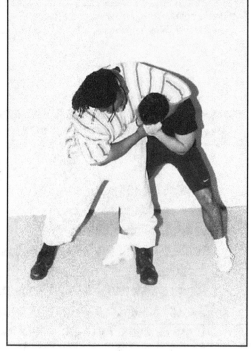

There are going to be times when you don't have the luxury of a fighting stance. Pictured here, the author is taken by surprise and placed in a side head lock.

Q: Are there any other stances that I should know about?

A: Yes. The first-strike stance, which is used prior to initiating a preemptive attack at your opponent. This deceptive self-defense posture facilitates "invisible deployment" of a preemptive strike while simultaneously protecting your vital targets against various possible counterattacks.

When assuming the first-strike stance, have both of your feet approximately shoulder width apart, knees slightly bent, with your body weight evenly distributed over each leg. Blade your body at a 45-degree angle from your adversary. This position will help situate your centerline at a protective angle from your opponent, enhance your balance, promote mobility, and set up your first-strike weapons. Next, make certain to keep your torso, pelvis, head, and back straight. And always stay relaxed and ready. Do not make the mistake of tensing your neck, shoulders, arms, or thighs. This muscular tension will most certainly throw off your timing, retard the speed of your movements, and telegraph your intentions.

Your hand positioning is another critical component of the first-strike stance. When

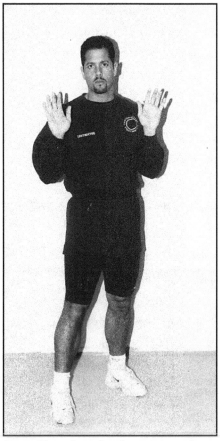

Pictured here, the author demonstrates a first strike stance used in the grappling range of hand to hand combat.

39

confronted with an opponent in the kicking and punching ranges of unarmed combat, keep both of your hands open, relaxed, and up to protect the upper gates of your centerline. Both of your palms should be facing the opponent with your lead arm bent between 90 and 120 degrees while your rear arm should be approximately 8 inches from your chin. When faced with an opponent in grappling range, keep both of your hands side by side of one another. Note: Remember that the only difference between a de-escalation stance and the first-strike stance is your intent.

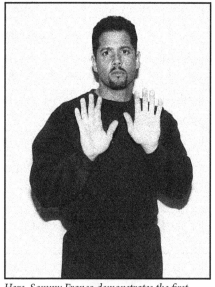

Here, Sammy Franco demonstrates the first strike stance for punching and kicking ranges.

HOW MANY DO YOU KNOW?

There are many stances used for reality-based self-defense. How many of these do you know?

- **Fighting stance**
- **De-escalation stance**
- **First right stance**
- **Natural stance**
- **Knife defense stance**
- **Bludgeon defense stance**
- **Stick fighting stance**
- **Firearm stances**

Hit First and Follow Up!

Q: Is it really all that important to hit my opponent first in a fight?

A: Yes. The fact of the matter is, the one who hits first will have a tremendous advantage in the fight. And when faced with a bigger and more powerful assailant, you want the greatest possible advantage. Striking first works especially well against larger opponents because most will not expect a smaller or weaker man to attack first.

Striking first permits you to neutralize your opponent swiftly while simultaneously negating his ability to retaliate. No time is wasted, and no unnecessary risks are taken. Moreover, it gives you the upper hand by allowing you to attack the adversary suddenly and unexpectedly. Hence, you demolish his defenses and ultimately take him out of the fight. An effective first strike is like a volatile explosion—it's a sudden and vehement outburst of destructive energy. In Chapter Four you will see how incredibly effective striking first can be.

Be careful! Successfully launching a first strike requires that you do not telegraph your intentions to your adversary. Clenching your teeth, widening your eyes, cocking your fist back, or tensing your shoulders are just a few telegraphic cues that will negate the element of surprise.

Q: But can I get into legal trouble if I hit my opponent first?

A: You can get into trouble if you are not legally justified to strike first. It is true that the most difficult aspect of delivering a first strike is determining exactly when you can strike first. Since every self-defense situation is different, there is no simple answer to this critical question. However, some fundamental elements must be present if you are going to legally launch a preemptive strike on your massive adversary.

First, you must never use force against another person unless it is absolutely justified. Force is broken down into two levels: lethal and nonlethal. Lethal force is defined as the amount of force that can cause serious bodily injury or death. Nonlethal force is defined as an amount of force that does not cause serious bodily injury or death.

Keep in mind that any time you use physical force against another person, you run the risk of having a civil suit filed against you. Anyone can hire a lawyer and sue for damages. Likewise, anyone can file a criminal complaint against you. Whether criminal charges will be brought against you depends upon the prosecutor's or grand jury's views of the facts. Nevertheless, I can tell you that if you are trained in the martial arts, you will be held to a much higher standard of behavior and conduct.

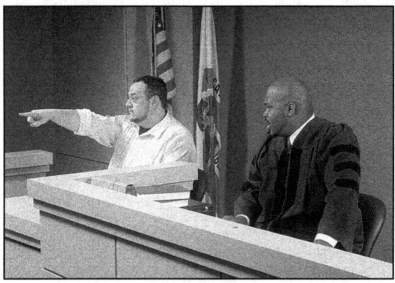

Any time you use physical force against another person (regardless of the size), you always run the risk of having a civil suit filed against you. Likewise, anyone can file a criminal complaint against you. When deciding to launch a first strike, be certain your actions are legally and morally justified in the eyes of the law.

Second, a first strike should only be used as an act of protection from unlawful injury or the immediate risk of unlawful injury. If you decide to launch a preemptive strike against your adversary, you must be certain that a reasonable threat exists and that it is absolutely necessary to protect yourself from immediate danger. Remember, the decision to launch a preemptive strike must always be a last resort where all other means of avoiding violence have been exhausted.

Q: Your first strike strategy makes sense, but what if my opponent attacks me first?

A: Your hulking adversary will undoubtedly have the immediate advantage, however, there are several defensive strategies and techniques that you can use to protect yourself. More will be discussed later in this chapter (see Defensive Considerations).

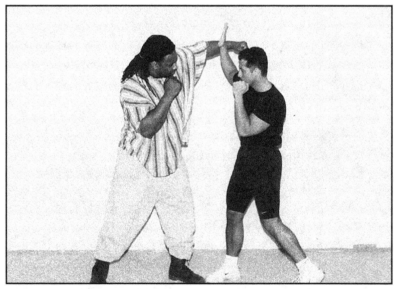

There's no escaping the fact that if your hulking adversary attacks first, he will have the immediate advantage over you. Luckily, there are several defensive tactics and strategies you can use to protect yourself.

The Bigger They Are, The Harder They Fall

Q: What do I do after I hit him with the first shot?

A: Good question. If your first strike doesn't incapacitate your adversary, and he still poses a reasonable threat, you must immediately follow up with secondary strikes. Essentially, secondary strikes are offensive techniques that comprise a compound attack. A compound attack is defined as two or more offensive strikes launched in strategic succession whereby you overwhelm your adversary with a flurry of full speed, full force blows.

Q: Do I always have to use a compound attack?

A: Only if your adversary still poses a reasonable threat to you or a loved one. If he does, you must employ a compound attack immediately following your first strike. Remember, the ultimate objective of a compound attack is to overwhelm your assailant by showering him with a barrage of rapid-fire blows designed to both injure him and demolish his defenses.

Explosiveness is a significant element of the compound attack. Your strikes and blows must be sudden, immediate, and exceedingly destructive. Your assault must never be progressive in nature—it must begin and end explosively.

Q: What about the strategy of tiring him out? For example, why can't I move around him and just pick him apart with jabs?

A: In a real-world self-defense situation, you must never "box" with your opponent. Do not dance around him throwing jabs. Remember, this is not a boxing match or a combat sport event. There is no time for that. You have to end the fight quickly and decisively. Anything less can spell disaster for you. This is especially important for people who study and practice mixed martial arts, boxing, and other sport oriented fighting styles.

Please understand that is not my intention to disparage or malign combat sports. I have a tremendous amount of respect for people who study these disciplines. However, it's my job to make it perfectly clear that many of the techniques used in sport competition can get you seriously injured and possibly killed in a street fight.

In street combat, it's critical that you always keep the offensive pressure on until your opponent is completely neutralized. Always remember that stagnating your "offensive flow", even for a second, will open you up to numerous dangers and risks.

The bottom line is that you must commit yourself 100 percent with the most effective flurry of blows appropriate to the ranges, angles, and use of force justification that presents itself.

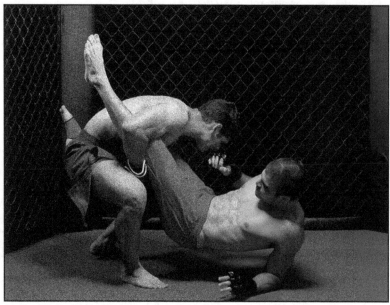

Many of the techniques used in sport competition can get you seriously injured and possibly killed in a street fight.

Q: What about the strategy of exploiting my opponent's fighting style?

A: That will not work either. The concept of exploiting your opponent's fighting style is a sparring and sport oriented strategy that cannot be effectively applied in a volatile street fight. A street fight is so fast and explosive that you will not have time to assess the opponent's reflexes or fighting style. In many ways, a street fight is likened to a car wreck!

Q: Okay, I think I understand what you are saying. So what exactly is an offensive flow?

A: The offensive flow is defined as continuous offensive movements (rapid-fire kicks, blows, and strikes) that ultimately neutralize your opponent.

Q: How do I keep the offensive flow going?

A: The key is not to disturb the fluidity of your strikes. If there is a pause during your barrage, your massive adversary can interrupt your compound attack by countering with a strike of his own or tackling you to the ground. Remember that the completion phase of your first strike should be the initiation phase of the second strike, and so on.

Target orientation and probable reaction dynamics also play important roles. Target orientation means having a workable knowledge of specific anatomical targets that are especially vulnerable in hand to hand combat. Probable reaction dynamics means understanding how your opponent will react to specific blows and strikes before they are ever delivered to their targets.

Q: Is there anything else I need to know about the compound attack?

A: Yes. Proper breathing is another substantial element of the compound attack. Here is one simple rule that should always be followed - exhale during the execution phase of your strike and inhale during its retraction phase. Never, ever hold your breath when delivering several consecutive blows. Doing so could lead to dizziness and fainting, among other possible complications.

Q: Why is time such a critical factor when delivering my compound attack?

A: The unfortunate fact is that your body can only sustain a compound attack for a short period of time. When engaged in a fight, your brain will quickly release adrenaline or epinephrine into your bloodstream, which will rapidly fuel your fighting and enhance your strength and power. This explosive boost of energy is commonly referred to as the *adrenaline dump*. However, your ability to exert to maintain this explosive effort in a compound attack will last no more than 30 to 60 seconds if you are above average shape. If the fight lasts longer than that, your strength and speed can drop by as much as 50 percent. The bottom line is every self-defense situation has to be one fast!

A close-up of the adrenaline molecule.

Q: Can you recommend any particular fighting combinations to use against a bigger dude?

A: Since every street fight is going to be different, there is no specific compound attack that you should employ against your opponent. However, in the upcoming chapters I'll give you a variety of compound attack scenarios that I have used in actual fights.

Mental Preparation

Q: How does the killer instinct factor into my fighting strategy?

A: If you want to defeat a massive and powerful adversary, then you must be savage. You must possess a combative mentality to channel a destructiveness exceeding that of your enemy. This mind-set is known as the killer instinct. The killer instinct is a vicious, combative mentality that surges to your consciousness and turns you into a vicious fighter who is free of fear, anger, and apprehension. It's a state of mind that permits you to fight to the best of your abilities.

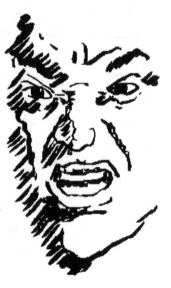

Q: So are you saying that I should try to "kill" my opponent in a fight?

A: The term "killer instinct" should not be taken literally. As a matter of fact, in many self-defense confrontations you will activate your killer instinct when only dispense intermediate use of force techniques. For the record, "killer instinct" does not necessarily refer to killing or terminating a criminal attacker.

Q: I read in your other books about the importance of pseudospeciation (assigning inferior qualities to your adversary) when fighting, but I find it difficult to do when I am faced with a larger opponent. What should I do?

A: You need to change your mind-set immediately. From a psychological perspective, you must not treat your massive adversary any differently than you would a smaller person. If you want to survive and ultimately prevail against a larger and stronger opponent on the streets, you must be a vicious beast.

When I say, "viciousness", I'm referring to a short-lived propensity to be extremely violent and destructive. Moreover, the only way to bring about this vicious intent is by pseudospeciating your enemy before and during the battle. By doing so, you will be able to unleash a controlled explosion of brutality without the constraints of moral or philosophical apprehension. However, you must be absolutely certain that your self-defense techniques are legally and morally justified in the eyes of the law.

Q: I still can't manage to get over the fear of fighting such a big person. Is there anything else I can do?

A: It's quite normal to experience fear. The important point is that you don't let fear turn into panic. Panic is an overpowering form of fear that can quickly cripple and immobilize you from protecting yourself or a loved one.

If you find yourself in a combat situation and you cannot control your fear, try to quickly convert your emotions into raw, vicious anger. Get mad! That's right: get pissed off at your opponent! This low-life piece of trash is going to injure or kill you or your loved one. Tear into him! I will be the first to admit that relying purely on anger is not the best way to defend yourself, but it can still serve as a powerful emotion that can be used in your favor.

Important Targets to Know About

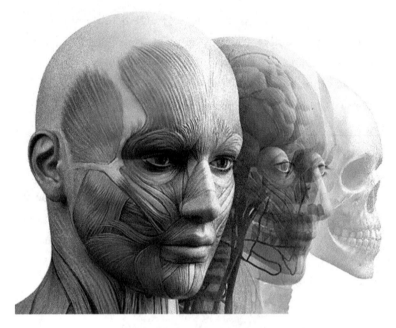

Q: Why do I have to know about human anatomy to win a street fight?

A: Anyone who is serious about winning a battle in the streets should have a fundamental understanding of human anatomy and physiology. Anatomy is the study of the body's structure, while physiology is the study of its function. Anatomical awareness is important because it provides you with target orientation; knowing exactly what anatomical targets to strike in a fight will make you an efficient technician that can get the job done quickly. Moreover, you need to know what vulnerable targets are presented on your own body that should be protected. Finally, as a combat specialist, you have a legal and moral responsibility to know what targets will stun, disfigure, cripple, or kill your hulking adversary.

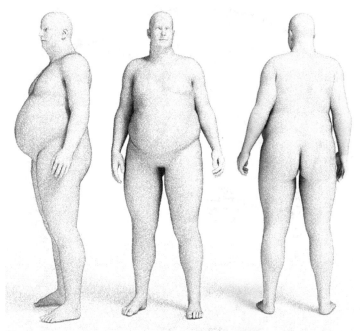

You don't have to be an anatomist to win a fight, but you must have a fundamental knowledge and understanding of human anatomy and physiology. This is especially important when fighting a larger adversary.

Q: Okay, so what are the best targets to strike on a larger adversary?

A: Through many years of study, training and actual fighting experience, I have concluded that there are essentially 13 "ideal" striking targets on the human body. They include: eyes, temples, nose, chin, back of neck, throat, solar plexus, ribs, testicles, thighs, knees, shins, instep/toes.

However, the best targets to strike on a large and powerful adversary are: the eyes, temple, nose, chin, throat, and knees.

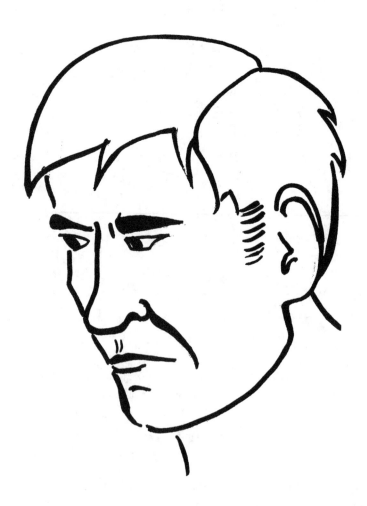

The majority of your primary targets will be located in the opponent's head region. This includes the eyes, temple, nose, chin, and throat.

THE EYES

The human eye is a very
complex and sophisticated organ
that lies within the bony socket of
the skull. Eyes are ideal targets to
attack because they are extremely
sensitive to the slightest touch.
Regardless of the opponent's

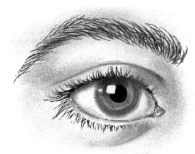

size, damaging his eyes will require very little force. You can scratch,
poke, and gouge the eyes from a variety of angles. Depending on the
force of your strike, eye strikes can cause temporary or permanent
blindness, extreme pain, rupture, shock, and unconsciousness.

THE TEMPLE

The temple is a very thin, weak
bone located on the side of the skull
approximately 1 inch from the eyes. Due
to its weak structure and proximity to the
brain, a powerful blow to this target can
be deadly. Other possible injuries include
unconsciousness, concussion, shock, and
coma.

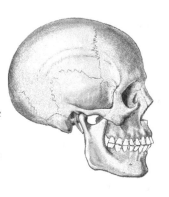

THE NOSE

The nose is constructed of thin bone,
cartilage, blood vessels and many nerves. It
is an excellent target because it can be struck
from three different directions (upward,
downward, and straight). A moderate blow can
cause stunning pain, watering eyes, temporary

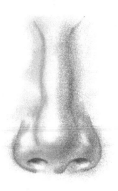

blindness, and hemorrhaging. A very forceful strike can result in shock and unconsciousness.

THE CHIN

The chin is another vulnerable target. When it is struck at a 45-degree angle, shock waves pulsate to the cerebellum and cerebral hemispheres of the brain, resulting in paralysis and unconsciousness. Other possible injuries can include a broken jaw, concussion, and whiplash.

THE THROAT

The throat is an especially vulnerable target because it is only protected by a thin layer of skin. The trachea, or windpipe, is a cartilaginous tube measuring approximately 4 1/2 inches in length and 1 inch in diameter. A powerful blow to this target can result in unconsciousness, blood drowning, massive hemorrhage, air starvation, and death.

THE KNEES

The knee is a very weak joint that is held together by a number of supporting ligaments. When the leg is locked and a forceful kick is delivered to the front of the joint, the cruciate ligaments will tear, resulting in excruciating pain,

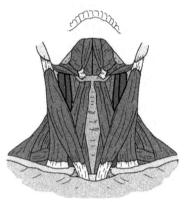

swelling, and immediate immobility.

Q: Why are these six targets the best ones to use against a larger adversary?

A: The eyes, temple, chin, nose, throat, and knees are ideal targets because neither muscle nor body fat can protect them from the force of your blows.

Q: Do I still need to know about the other seven targets?

A: Yes. While the eyes, temple, chin, nose, throat, and knees are your primary targets, the other seven anatomical targets (back of neck, solar plexus, ribs, testicles, thighs, shins, and instep/toes) are important as well.

Q: What are reaction dynamics and why is it important in a street fight?

A: Reaction dynamics is simply the opponent's physical response to the impact of your blows and strikes. A thorough understanding of general reaction dynamics is important because it will allow you to exploit your opponent's openings and maintain an effective compound attack. If you want to get a bird's eye view of various reaction dynamics, see Chapter Four.

Q: Will a large man have the same reaction dynamics as his smaller counterpart?

A: Yes, as long as you hit him hard enough. As I mentioned earlier, because of the opponent's size and bodyweight, his bones are going to be larger and thicker and he will be able to take greater punishment. If he's significantly overweight, his body fat will act as a shield that protects his muscles and nerves from the force and impact of your blows.

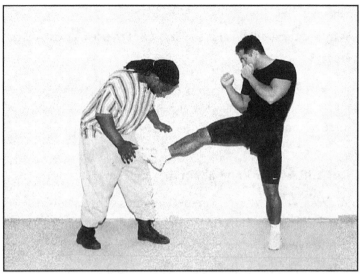

If you want to maintain the offensive flow in a fight, you better have a sound understanding of the opponents reaction dynamics. Notice how the impact of the basic push kick will cause the opponent to fall forward and drop is hands-down. You must learn how to exploit this opening.

Q: Is it okay to "head-hunt"?

A: Strategically attacking the opponent's head, or "head-hunting," is a very effective street-fighting strategy that has proven its effectiveness time and time again. Nevertheless, it may be difficult to do when fighting an opponent of appreciable height. The best advice I can give you is to simply use your best judgment during the fight. If the head presents itself as a target, go for it!

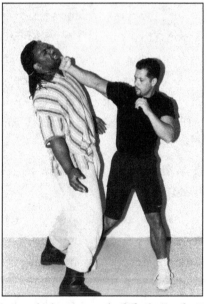

Because of his superior height, a taller opponents had targets can be difficult to strike. In this photo, author Sammy Franco just barely connects with his hook punch.

Fighting Ranges

Q: What is range proficiency and why is it so important when fighting a large adversary?

A: Since a large and powerful adversary is more likely to rush through the ranges of combat with reckless abandon, it behooves you to be range proficient. Range proficiency means that you have the skill and ability to effectively fight your adversary from all three distances of unarmed combat. Here is a quick breakdown of the three ranges. Commit them to memory!

Kicking range: At this distance, you are usually too far away to strike with your hands, so you would use your legs to strike your adversary. For real-life combat, you should only employ low-line kicks. These kicks are directed to targets below the assailant's waist, such as the groin, thigh, knee joint, and shinbone.

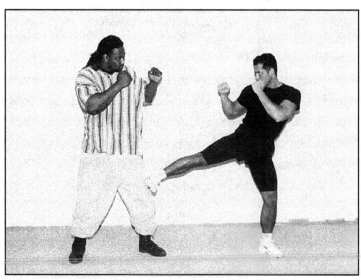

The kicking distance of unarmed combat.

Punching range: This is the midrange of unarmed combat. At this distance, you are close enough to your assailant to strike him with your hands. Hand strikes do not require as much room as kicking, and the surface you are standing on is not as critical a concern.

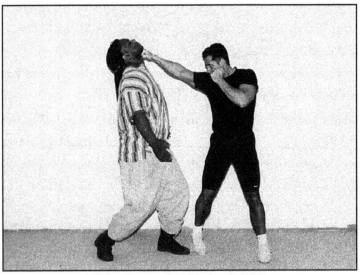

The punching range of unarmed combat.

Grappling range: The third and closest range of unarmed combat is the grappling range. At this distance, you are too close to your adversary to kick or execute most hand strikes, so you would use close-quarter tools and techniques to neutralize your assailant. Grappling range is divided into two planes. The vertical plane is where you are standing toe-to-toe with your assailant. The horizontal plane is where you and the enemy are ground fighting.

Q: What is the neutral zone?

A: The neutral zone is the distance at which neither you nor your opponent can strike or kick each other. It is not a range of unarmed combat.

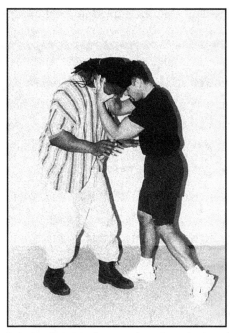

The grappling range (vertical plane) of unarmed combat. Also known as clinch range.

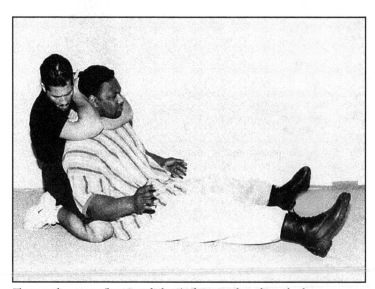

The grappling range (horizontal plane) of unarmed combat. Also known as ground fighting.

Q: Why is the neutral zone an important part of my overall fighting strategy?

A: The strategic implication of the neutral zone is that it creates distance between you and your monstrous adversary. This, in turn, will allow you to temporarily assess your assailant and choose the appropriate tactical response. If your adversary attacks first, it will also provide you with enhanced reaction time so that you can protect yourself adequately. Beware, however, because not all assailants, situations, or environments will afford you the luxury of maintaining a neutral zone.

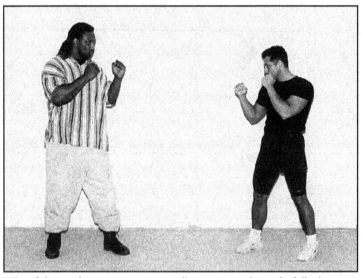

When fighting a bigger opponent, a smaller person needs to take full advantage of his defensive space. Pictured here, the neutral zone of unarmed combat.

Q: What is the preferred range of combat when fighting a larger man?

A: From a first-strike perspective the punching range is preferred, because your adversary's defensive reaction time will be reduced. Unlike the kicking range, you can efficiently deliver a flurry of full-speed blows in the punching range. Most importantly, compared to the grappling range, the punching range requires only moderate bodily commitment.

Q: What is the least preferred range of combat when fighting a larger man?

A: The grappling range in the horizontal plane. More will be explained in Chapter Five.

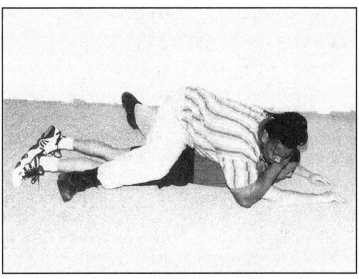

When fighting an adversary of any size, the least preferred range of unarmed combat is grappling in the horizontal plane. In this photo, the larger man takes full advantage of his size and weight.

Stay on Your Feet and Keep Moving

Q: Why is explosive footwork important when fighting a larger adversary?

A: In offense, explosive footwork can be a major asset, allowing you to maintain the offensive flow. In defense, it allows you to disengage quickly from a range of overwhelming assaults. In some instances, explosive footwork will help you acquire superior positioning. Finally, and most importantly, it is a natural power generator that will enhance the overall power of your blows.

Q: How do I develop explosive footwork?

A: Explosive footwork is structured around four general directions: advancing, retreating, moving right, and moving left. Practice the following movements slowly in front of a full-length mirror until your actions are quick and natural.

Moving forward (advance): From your stance, move your front foot forward (approximately 18-24 inches) and then advance your rear foot an equal distance.

Moving backward (retreat): From your stance, move your rear foot backward (approximately 18-24 inches) and then move your front foot an equal distance.

Moving right (sidestep right): From your stance, move your right foot to the right (approximately 18-24 inches) and then move your left foot an equal distance.

Moving left (sidestep left): From your stance, move your left foot to the left (approximately 18-24 inches) and then move your right foot an equal distance.

Once you have grasped the fundamentals of footwork, you can practice various footwork drills. For example, start by assuming a good fighting stance and then have your training partner call out various direction commands (advance, move right, switch your stance, etc.) at various cadences. Make certain to maintain proper stance form throughout the course of the exercise. You can also wear a weighted vest to further strengthen and condition your leg muscles.

Q: What is the difference between sidestepping and strategic circling?

A: Both sidestepping and strategic circling are essential components of footwork. Generally, sidestepping is used for defensive purposes to evade an opponent's attack, whereas strategic circling can be used to evade an attack and immediately counter the adversary.

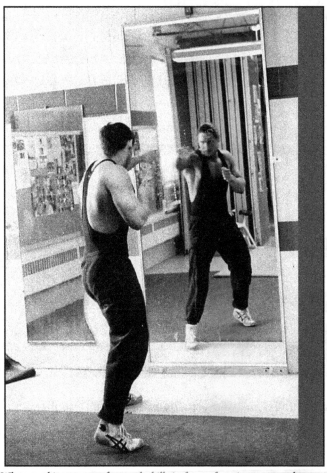

When working on your footwork skills in front of a mirror, remember to maintain good form and always keep both of your hands up.

Q: What is the difference between "step and lift" and "step and drag" footwork?

A.   Step and lift footwork is your primary method of mobility, and it is performed by moving the foot closest to the direction that you want to go first, and letting the other foot follow an equal distance. Since both of your feet are being lifted off the ground, it should be used when you are standing on stable terrain.

Lifting one foot quickly off the ground and dragging the other behind is called step and drag footwork. It is the most sure-footed method of stepping and it is most often used when you are forced to fight an enemy on slippery and unstable terrain, such as ice, snow, wet surfaces, sand, gravel, mulch, mud, and rock.

Don't look at the ground!

One of the most common mistakes made when performing footwork drills in front of a mirror is to look at the floor. Avoid this bad habit! Remember, in a street fight, you want to keep your eyes on your opponent, not the ground.

Q: What is the relocation principle and how is it applied?

A: The relocation principle is quite simple. After you unleash your compound attack, immediately move to a new location by flanking your enemy. Based on the principles of strategic movement and surprise, relocating dramatically enhances your safety by making it difficult for your adversary to identify your position after you have injured him. Keep in mind that if your opponent does not know exactly where you are, he will not be able to effectively counterattack. Also bear in mind that relocating can mean fleeing from the fight altogether.

Defensive Considerations

Q: When defending against a larger opponent, why should I be concerned about his "inside position"?

A: From a defensive perspective, the opponent's inside position (the area between both of his arms) is very dangerous because it's where he has the greatest amount of strength, leverage, and control. The inside position allows your opponent to leverage both his center of gravity and body weight to his full advantage. It's also where he can launch his natural body weapons (i.e., punches, elbow and knee strikes, etc.) with ease.

If you find yourself in a situation where you have to defend against your opponent, try to maneuver yourself to the outside of his inside position. This will require quick footwork in conjunction with proper timing.

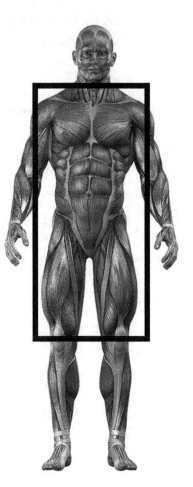

The inside position is the area between the opponent's arms. From a defensive perspective, this is the most dangerous area for you.

Don't be defensive!

Never approach unarmed combat defensively, especially when faced with a bigger opponent. A defensive fighter is someone who allows his adversary the opportunity to seize and maintain offensive control. Be careful! This defensive mindset can get you killed in the real world.

Q: What should my biggest concern be when defending against a larger and stronger adversary?

A: There are two major concerns that you should have when defending against a massive adversary. First, you must be aware that a larger and stronger opponent is most likely going to use his mass and strength to overwhelm you. He might do this by rushing and tackling you to the floor or by simply placing you in a bear hug and squeezing the life out of you.

Second, if he swings at you, there's always the risk of losing your balance when blocking his weighty punches. Since a larger and stronger adversary can generate tremendous force when executing circular blows (e.g., hook punches and haymakers), you can easily be knocked off balance. This disruption in balance will most likely impede your ability to counterattack.

Q: If blocking a powerful swing can knock me off balance, what about bobbing and weaving as a defensive response?

A: The bob and weave is dangerous because it exposes you to a possible knee or elbow strike. Moreover, the bob and weave lacks economy of motion. And if you misjudge the height of the opponent's swing, you can move your head right into the path of the blow. Stick to blocking. It is much safer!

Q: When blocking a punch, is there anything I can do to prevent myself from being thrown off balance?

A: It is imperative that you maintain a strong center of balance. This can be accomplished by utilizing a solid fighting stance and maintaining a 50-percent weight distribution. This "noncommittal" weight distribution will provide you with the necessary stability to withstand and defend powerful blows and strikes. Also, when extending your blocking arm, be certain to maximally increase your trunk rotation and set your feet firmly in the ground.

Keep Your Balance!

Losing your balance is one of the greatest concerns when defending against a larger and stronger foe. Always maintain a solid and stable stance when defending against his assault.

Q: What blocks do I have to know if I am going to fight a bigger person?

A: There are just four blocks that you need to know. They are: high blocks, mid blocks, elbow blocks, and leg blocks.

High block: The high block is used to defend against overhead blows. To execute the lead high block, simply raise your lead arm up and extend your forearm out and above your head. Be careful not to position your arm where your head is exposed. Make certain your hand is open and not clenched. The mechanics for the lead high block are the same for the rear high block. Raise your rear arm up and extend your forearm out and above your head.

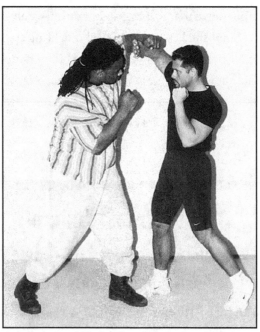

A properly timed block will work every time. In this photo, Sammy Franco uses a high block to intercept his opponents forceful punch.

Mid block: The mid block is used against circular blows to your head or upper torso. To perform the block, raise either your right or left arm up at approximately 90 degrees while simultaneously pronating it into the direction of the strike. Make contact with the belly of your forearm at the assailant's wrist or forearm and keep your hand open to increase the surface area of your block.

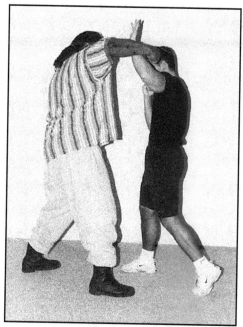

The most common punch thrown in a fight is the right hook or haymaker. Here, the author uses a mid block to defend against the attack.

Elbow block: The elbow block is used to intercept circular blows to your midsection, such as uppercuts, shovel hooks, and even hook kicks. To execute the elbow block, drop your elbow down and simultaneously twist your body toward your centerline. Be certain to keep your elbow perpendicular to the floor and keep your hands relaxed and close to your chest.

Leg block: The leg block is used to intercept, choke, or deflect an oncoming kick. It can be delivered from either your lead or rear leg, and it can be positioned at a variety of different angles, heights, and vantages. Generally, the leg block should be used only when you cannot evade the opponent's attack. NOTE: the leg block can also be used to evade a foot-sweep technique.

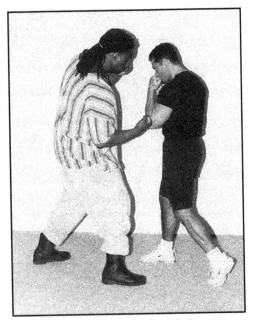

Pictured here, the elbow block.

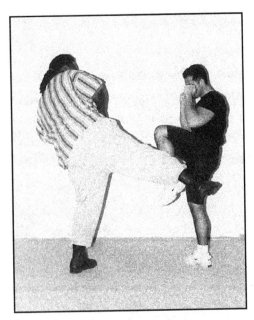

Pictured here, the leg block.

Q: Can you recommend any drills for developing my blocking skills?

A: Actually, there are two. The solo blocking drill is used to sharpen and refine your basic blocking technique without the pressure of timing. Begin by assuming a fighting stance in front of a full-length mirror. Then, slowly execute a high block, noting any flaws in the execution of the movement, alternating right and left arms, and returning to the starting position. Next, execute a mid block at moderate speed, noting any mistakes in the execution of the movement, alternating right and left arms, and returning to the starting position. Finally, execute an elbow block at moderate speed, noting any flaws in the execution of the movement, alternating right and left arms, and returning to the starting position. Keep in mind that the solo blocking drill can also be conducted with the eyes closed to develop a kinesthetic feel for the technique.

The 360-degree blocking drill is another excellent exercise for developing your blocking skills. Begin by positioning yourself in a 45-degree stance (with your arms up) with your training partner standing approximately three feet from you. Next, have your training partner deliver a series of random swings at your head or torso while you immediately respond with the appropriate blocks. As you become more proficient with this drill, your training partner should deliver a sequence of random swings while moving in various directions. **Caution:** Remember to start out slowly and progressively build up the speed and force of your strikes.

Q: What is the best way to defend against straight blows?

A: Parrying. The parry is a quick, forceful slap that redirects your opponent's linear strike (jabs, straights, etc.). Two types of parries need to be mastered: horizontal and vertical. Both can be executed from the right and left hands.

Horizontal parry: To properly execute a horizontal parry, begin in a fighting stance and move your lead hand horizontally across your body (centerline) to deflect and redirect the assailant's punch. Immediately return to your guard position. When parrying, be certain to make contact with the palm of your hand and keep your thumb married to the side of your hand. With sufficient training, you can effectively incorporate the horizontal parry with your slipping maneuvers.

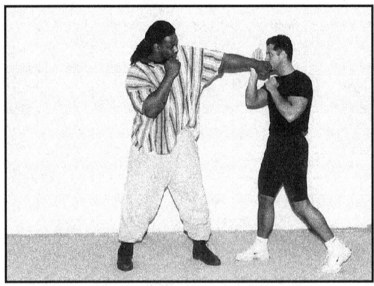

The author demonstrates a right hand horizontal parry.

Vertical parry: To execute a vertical parry, begin in a stance and move your hand vertically down your body (centerline) to deflect and redirect the assailant's blow. Again, do not forget to counterattack your assailant.

A word of caution: Do not parry with your fingers. The fingers are structurally weak, and they can be jammed or broken easily. In addition, never attempt to parry a hook punch, or any circular blow for that matter. A parry simply does not have the "structural integrity" to stop the blow. Instead, use a mid block to defend against the hook punch.

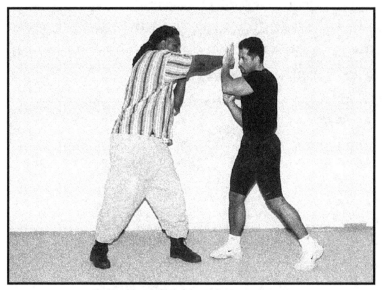

Pictured here, the left hand horizontal parry.

Q: Is parrying the only way to defend against straight punches?

A: No, slipping is another effective method. Slipping is a quick defensive maneuver that permits you to avoid an assailant's linear blow without stepping out of range. Safe and effective slipping requires precise timing and is accomplished by quickly snapping the head and upper torso sideways (right or left) or backward to avoid the oncoming blow. Keep in mind that one of the greatest advantages to slipping is that it frees your hands so you can simultaneously counter your attacker. There are three ways to slip. They include the following maneuvers:

Slipping right: Start from a stance and quickly sway your head and upper torso to the right to avoid the assailant's blow. Quickly counter or return to the starting position.

Slipping left: Start from a stance and quickly sway your head and upper torso to the left to avoid the assailant's linear blow. Quickly counter or return to the starting position.

Slipping back (also called the snap back): Start from a stance and quickly snap your head back enough to avoid being hit. Quickly counter or return to the starting position.

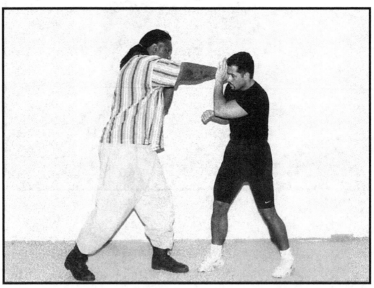

Here, Sammy Franco simultaneously slips and parries his opponent's punch.

Q: Are there any drills I can do to develop my parrying and slipping skills?

A: Yes. The parrying drill is designed to sharpen both your parrying and slipping skills. Start out by positioning yourself in a fighting stance with your training partner standing approximately 3 feet from you. Next, have your partner deliver a series of straight blows (at moderate speed) directed toward your head and torso and respond with the appropriate parry. Remember to make contact with the palm of your hand. Continue this drill for approximately 30 seconds and then switch places with your partner. In addition, you can incorporate slipping maneuvers into the drill. Just remember to start out slowly and progressively build up speed and intensity.

Q: I always forget to keep my chin down when fighting. Is there anything you can recommend to help me break this bad habit?

A: Try shadow fighting with a chalkboard eraser or a thick sponge under your chin. This is a simple and effective way to remind you to keep your chin angled down when fighting.

Q: Can you tell me some common mistakes made when fighting?

A: Here are a few:

- Failing to move when defending
- Not keeping your hands up
- Not keeping your elbows in
- Retreating instead of sidestepping.

Q: What is the biggest mistake I can make when defending against a larger and stronger opponent?

A: Closing your eyes or reflexively dropping your head when being bombarded with blows—also known as the "ostrich defense"—can get you killed in a street fight. With the ostrich defense, the practitioner will look away from that which he fears (punches, kicks, and strikes) in hopes that it will go away. His reasoning is, *"If I can't see it, it can't hurt me."*

One of the best ways to prevent the ostrich defense is to practice the hip-fusing drill (described in the next chapter) while making a conscious effort to keep your head erect and your eyes open amid flying blows. If you are hit, do not panic. Just keep moving, maintain proper breathing, apply the appropriate defensive response, and counterattack when the opportunity presents itself.

Q: Is there anything I can do to improve my reaction time in a fight?

A: Yes. First, read advance information about your opponent's attack by watching his body language. I call this telegraphic cognizance. For example, when your adversary shifts his shoulders back, you know he's about to deliver a punch.

Second, limit your number of defensive responses to a particular type of attack. For example, if your adversary attacks with a straight blow to your head, you should have only one specific defensive response programmed. In this instance, you would use a parry to redirect the blow.

Third, all of your defensive responses should be natural and executed in a simple fashion. Again, in the case of the straight blow, not only would you execute a parry, but you would also situate it on the same side of the opponent's punch (this is referred to as mirror-image parrying).

Fourth, your defensive responses must be practiced repeatedly until they become second nature. Employ the different blocking and parrying drills that I discussed earlier and you will noticeably improve.

Q: What if my opponent tackles me to the ground? What then?

A: Since there is a very good chance that this can occur, I have devoted an entire chapter to this subject. See Chapter 5 for more information.

The Game Plan - Putting everything together!

Q: So exactly what is my battle plan when fighting a larger and stronger adversary?

A: There are 10 strategic points to bear in mind:

1)   Stay calm and relaxed. Don't let him psych you out!

2)   Wait in the neutral zone until you are ready to attack.

3)   When the opportunity presents itself, strike first and strike fast!

4)   Hit the opponent as hard as possible, utilizing all your power generators.

5)   Exploit his reaction dynamics with a vicious compound attack.

6)   Stay on your feet, maintain the offensive flow, and do not give him the ability to grab hold of you.

7)   Be cognizant of your range and do not let him restrict your mobility.

8)   Once the opponent is incapacitated, move to a safe location.

9)   Do everything in your power to avoid a ground fight.

10) If you screw up, keep fighting. Never, ever give up!

Q: Is there anything else I need to know before moving on to the next chapter?

A: No. You now have a precise battle plan that you can take with you to the streets.

The Bigger They Are, The Harder They Fall

Chapter Three
Preparing for the Beast

"In peace, as a wise man, he should make suitable preparation for war."   *-Horace (65-8 B.C)*

Now it's time to look into training. In this chapter, I'll show you how to systematically develop the skills and attributes necessary to defeat a massive opponent in a street fight. Since you are at such a size disadvantage, it is imperative that you take the time to train and condition your body for the rigors of street combat. There is no way around it!

Basic Training

Q: What type of training do I need to do?

A: First and foremost, your training must be combat oriented. Everything you do must specifically relate to the sobering realities of a vicious street fight. Your skills and techniques must be efficient, effective, safe, and capable of being applied under "real-world" conditions against a larger and stronger opponent.

Above all, if you want to be capable of fight and ultimately defeat a massive adversary, stay away from sport and ritual-oriented martial arts training. Remember, you are not training for the octagon or boxing ring. You are training for something much more dangerous - the streets!

In this book, I have designed a combat-oriented program that is divided into four general categories. They are:

The Bigger They Are, The Harder They Fall

- *Mental training*
- *Cardiovascular training*
- *Weight training*
- *Equipment training*

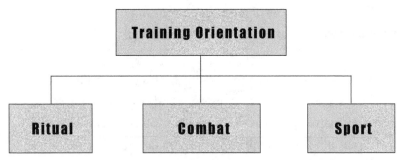

There are three types of training orientations: ritual, combat, and sport. Reality-based self-defense training focuses exclusively on combat oriented training.

Q: What elements are necessary for a good combat-oriented training program?

A: First, you need to be consistent with your training. You need to have a realistic training regimen and stick to it, no matter what. This will require a considerable amount of discipline on your part.

The second element is motivation. While strong motivation is common in students just launching into the study of self-defense, the challenge is to sustain that level and, in fact, increase motivation and desire as time goes on.

Even with motivation there is the risk of frustration in the early phases of self-defense and combat training. However, once you start to develop the basic skills, you may be surprised to see gains come in leaps and bounds. The bottom line is, if you want it bad enough, you will make it happen.

Q: Do I really have to warm up before working out?

A: Yes. Warming up before a workout is important for several reasons. It safely increases your heart rate, significantly reduces the possibility of muscle and tendon strain, and sets the proper frame of mind for your workout.

Q: What are the best exercises for warming up?

A: Jumping jacks, rope skipping, light shadow fighting, and stretching. Actually, stretching is one of the most important warm-up exercises that you can perform. Stretching increases your flexibility and agility and minimizes muscle tears. Remember that a flexible muscle reacts and contracts faster than a nonflexible muscle, which means improved combative performance.

Here are a few good stretches that you should add to your training regimen. Remember to hold each stretch for a minimum of 30 seconds, breathe normally, and avoid any bouncing movements.

Neck turns: Turn your head to the right side, stretching your chin toward your right shoulder. Turn your head back to the center and repeat to the left side.

Shoulder stretch: Stand with your feet approximately shoulder width apart. Slowly raise your right arm overhead and stretch as far as you can without bending your torso.

Repeat with your left arm.

Forearm stretch: Extend your right arm in front of you with your palm facing downward. With your left hand, grasp the fingers of your right hand and pull back slowly, stretching the forearm. Repeat the same stretch with your left arm.

Triceps stretch: Raise your right arm straight up, so your upper arm is close to your ear. Bend at the elbow, and let your right hand fall to the back of your neck. With your left arm, reach behind your head and place your hand on top of the bent elbow. Gently pull down and back on the elbow. Repeat with other arm.

Trunk stretch: Stand with your feet approximately shoulder width apart. Stretch your left arm over your head and slowly bend to the right. Repeat on the opposite side.

Chest stretch: Stand with your feet approximately shoulder width apart. Clasp your hands behind your back and gently press your arms upward while keeping your arms straight.

Back stretch: Lie on your back and bring your right knee to your chest. Hold your knee with both hands and slowly pull in. Repeat with the other knee.

Lower back reach: Sit on the floor with your legs straight in front of you. Reach forward toward your toes, keeping your head up and lower back slightly arched. Avoid rounding your back. Breathe normally and hold for a count of 30.

Butterfly stretch: Sit on the floor, bend your knees to the sides, and bring the soles of your feet together. Place your hands on your knees and gently press your knees toward the floor. Remember to keep your back straight.

Hamstring stretch: Stand with your right foot crossed over the left. Bend at the hips, reaching toward the floor and keeping your knees slightly bent. Repeat with the opposite foot.

Leaning calf stretch: Stand about 2 1/2 feet from a wall. Place your hands on the wall and lean in, gently pushing your hips forward. Keep both of your legs straight and heels flat on the floor.

Standing calf stretch: Stand with your feet together. Extend your right leg in front of you and place your heel on the floor with your toes in the air. While keeping your back straight, bend forward at the hips until you feel the stretch in your right calf. Repeat with the left leg.

Quadriceps stretch: From a standing position, reach back to grasp your right ankle with your right hand. Pull the heel of your foot toward your buttocks. You may need to place your other hand on the wall for balance and support. Repeat with your left leg.

Are you a Risk Taker?

Combat requires taking risks, but you can reduce those risks by through proper planning and methodical training.

Q: Should I train every day?

A: No. You will burn out. Resting the body is an important element of self-defense/combat training. Working out day after day will undoubtedly lead to over training or injury. The body needs time to recoup and rebuild itself from grueling workouts.

Q: How do I know if I am over training and what are some of the symptoms?

A: Some symptoms of burn-out include physical illness,

boredom, anxiety, disinterest in training, poor physical performance, general sluggish behavior, and fatigue.

Self-Mastery is Your Goal!

Mastery of the mind, body and spirit is the core essence of combat training.

Q: Do you have any suggestions that will help me avoid burning out?

A: Here are a few tips to help avoid over training and burn-out:

• Make your workouts intense but enjoyable.

• Stagger the intensity of your workouts.

• Work out while listening to different types of music.

• Pace yourself during your workouts—don't try to do it all in one day.

• Listen to your body—if you don't feel up to working out, then skip a day.

• Work out in different types of environments.

• Use different types of training equipment.

• Work out with different training partners.

• Keep accurate records of your training routine.

• Vary the intensity of your training in your workout.

• Monitor your mental and physical energy levels daily.

Q: Should I train with a partner?

A: Yes. A good training partner will motivate, challenge, and push you to your limits. When weight training with heavy poundage, a training partner can spot you and force out those extra repetitions. Furthermore, you will need a partner to hold and manipulate some of the training equipment (focus mitts, striking shield, kicking cylinder, etc.). Caution: while a good training partner can be a big help, having a bad one can be disastrous. So, be careful who you choose.

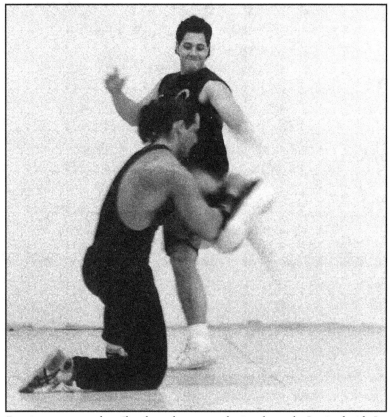

Even in my younger days, I've always been very selective about who I trained with. In this photograph, my training partner holds the kicking pads with all of his might.

Q: Is there anything I can do to increase the intensity of my workouts?

A: Yes. Train to the sounds of hard-driving rock music. Not only will your physical performance improve, but also your mental attitude will be enhanced dramatically.

MORE COMBAT TRAINING TIPS

- Train for the street, not the ring.
- Don't wear gis or other classic martial arts uniforms.
- Don't train barefoot, wear shoes.
- Don't be submission oriented - be destruction oriented.
- Emphasize contact oriented drills and exercises.
- Practice efficient, effective, and safe techniques designed for real-world self-defense situations.
- Try to evaluate your performance after every workout.
- Listen carefully to your training partner's comments and observations.
- Assess the combat utility behind every drill you perform.
- Always maintain a "hard-core" yet positive attitude.

Q: Do you have any other suggestions about training?

A: Yes. Always be cognizant of your training objective. In this case, you are looking to defeat a larger and stronger adversary in a real-life combat situation. Therefore, you should be developing practical and efficient skills that will help you survive this life-threatening encounter.

Mental Training

Q: What mental exercises can I do to prepare myself for a larger and stronger adversary?

A: Mental visualization should be a regular part of your training routine. Visualization is the purposeful formation of mental images to improve both your training and combative performance. As a training aid, it will enhance your cardiovascular and weight-lifting sessions. Moreover, it helps keep you motivated during those grueling equipment-training workouts.

On a combat level, mental visualization improves your assessment skills and general reaction time, develops sharper psycho-motor skills, and helps crystallize your killer instinct.

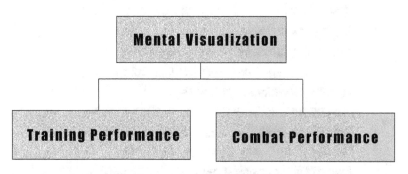

Mental visualization is used for improving both training and combat performance.

Q: Can you give me a few examples of what I should visualize?

A: Sure. Three times per week, mentally rehearse strategic solutions to various street-fighting scenarios. For example, move your Herculean adversary into different ranges of combat, select appropriate anatomical targets and attack combinations, and visualize your assailant's possible reaction dynamics from specific strikes and blows. Alternatively, try scrutinizing the five tactical options (comply, escape, de-escalate, assert, and fight back) as they relate to a variety of possible street-fighting scenarios. However, bear in mind that if you are to truly benefit from visualization exercises, your images must always be crystal clear.

INCLUDE THESE IMPORTANT FACTORS WHEN VISUALIZING COMBAT SCENARIOS

- Opponent's physical characteristics: height, weight, etc.
- Opponent's approximate age
- Opponent's deformities
- Opponent's ethnicity or race
- Opponent's accent (if any) and what he is saying to you
- Opponent's clothing
- Opponent's intent and general demeanor
- Opponent's range and positioning from you
- Opponent's weapon capability
- The location: bar, city street, dark alley, parking lot, etc.
- The smells, sounds, taste, and feel of the environment
- The year, month, day, and hour of the fight
- Your strategic assessment of the immediate situation
- Your level of confidence from a third person perspective
- Your intent and objective (prior to and during combat)
- Your first strike technique
- The opponents reaction dynamics to your first strike as well as your secondary blows.
- Your mental state after the fight
- Your physical state after the fight

Cardiovascular Training

Q: What are two of the best cardiovascular exercises for street self-defense?

A: Rope skipping, wind sprints and running.

Q: How will rope skipping help me in a street fight?

A: Skipping rope on a regular basis will make you quick and light on your feet during a fight. This is particularly important when fighting a larger opponent. Jumping rope also conditions your heart and enhances your coordination, endurance, balance, and agility.

Q: I am not that coordinated. Can you give me some tips when skipping?

A: Yes. First, relax your arms and shoulders when jumping. Second, remember to push off your toes and land gently on the balls of your feet. Third, keep your elbows close to your sides and use your wrists and forearms to turn the rope. Fourth, keep your head up, maintain good posture, and bend naturally at the knees and hips. Also, remember to jump low—approximately 1 inch off the ground.

The Bigger They Are, The Harder They Fall

Q: Why is running recommended?

A: Running is one of the most effective methods of conditioning your cardiovascular system for the harsh demands of street fighting. It improves wind capacity, endurance, circulation, and muscle tone. Running strengthens the legs, burns a significant amount of calories, and will stimulate the metabolism (a vital component of weight management). Running is also an ideal time to practice mental visualization.

All of your running sessions should start with a brisk jog, ultimately working up to a faster pace. Remember to start slowly and progressively build up speed. Make it your goal to run a minimum of three times per week for a duration of approximately 30-50 minutes.

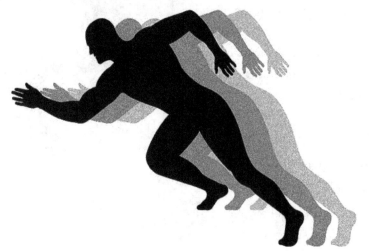

Wind sprints are great for improving your speed, aerobic capacity and combat explosiveness.

Q: How far should I sprint?
A: Much will depend on your current level of conditioning. Some people will find a 40 meter sprint challenging while others will require greater distances. Frankly, there is no standard distance. Experiment and see what distance works best for you.

Q: When is the best time to run?

A: In the morning the air is usually cleaner and cooler.

Q: What is the best surface to run on?

A: Short grass is the best surface to run on. Compared to concrete and asphalt, running on the grass minimizes the pressure and strain on your shins and knees.

Q: I sometimes get bored when I run. Do you have any suggestions?

A: Try mixing it up. Try running laps around the track, switch to jogging or walking with a weight vest, or run up and down stadium steps or bleachers. You are only limited buyer own imagination. You can also add music to your workouts. Listening to powerful and aggressive tunes will psyche you up and push you to your physical limits during a grueling run.

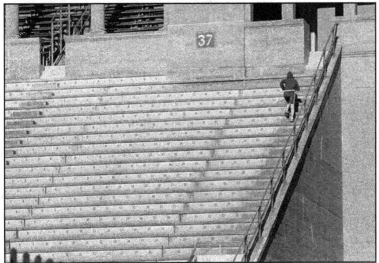

There are many benefits of running stadium stairs or bleachers. Some include: increased speed and endurance, improved leg strength, improved cardiovascular health, and combat explosiveness.

Weight Training

Q: Besides working on my fighting skills, is there anything else I can do to physically prepare myself for a larger opponent?

A: Yes. Hit the weights hard! A serious weight-training program combined with consistent stretching exercises is important. The bottom line is that you need to strengthen your bones and muscles to withstand the rigors of street combat, especially when you are fighting a larger and stronger opponent.

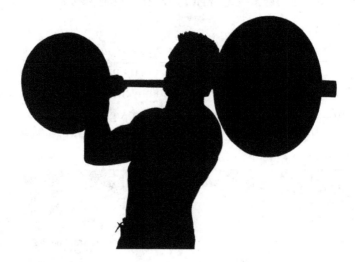

Q: I really don't know much about weight training. What are some of the basic principles?

A: There are four general principles that form the foundation of an effective weight-training program. First, an effective weight-training program must progressively overload your muscles. Second, as your muscles become stronger, the resistance must be increased. Third, strength and size gains come quicker from fewer reps and heavy weights. Fourth, your muscles must be given sufficient time to recuperate from training.

When weight training, be certain to maintain proper form and execute all your movements in a smooth and controlled fashion. If you are unfamiliar with a particular exercise, please see my book *War Machine: How to Transform Yourself into a Vicious and Deadly Street Fighter.*

Q: Exactly which exercises will help me fight a larger and stronger opponent?

A: There are many, however, here are just a few staple exercises that should be included in your program. They include:

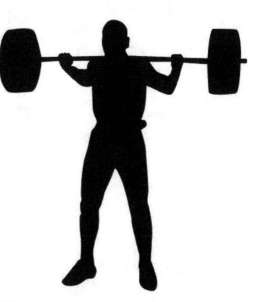

- **Bench press**
- **Pull-ups**
- **Deadlifts**
- **Squats**
- **Military press**
- **Bicep curls**
- **Hammer curls**
- **Barbell shrugs**
- **Dips**
- **Sit-ups**

Q: Do you recommend taking supplements when weight training?

A: I most certainly do. Throughout the years, I have discovered three supplements that are tried and true for gaining lean muscle mass and strength. They include: creatine, glutamine and whey protein.

Creatine is a tasteless and odorless, white powder that is relatively inexpensive. It actually mimics some of the effects of anabolic steroids. While results will vary from person to person, it's not uncommon for some people to gain 5 to 10 pounds of lean muscle within a few weeks of intense weight training.

Glutamine is an amino acid that plays a vital role in protein synthesis, prevention of muscle breakdown, and the secretion of human growth hormone.

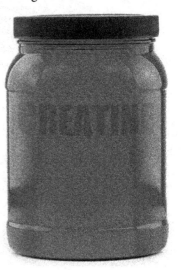

Whey is a high quality protein that is loaded with all the essential amino acids. The benefit to whey protein include: building muscle mass, maintaining muscle tone, increased strength, and the improvement of overall combat performance.

Equipment Training

Q: What type of equipment do you recommend for combat training?

A: There are several pieces of equipment that you should use. They include the heavy bag, body opponent bag (BOB), double-end bag, focus mitts, striking shield, and kicking cylinder. Let's look at each one.

The Heavy Bag

The heavy bag is the best piece of equipment for developing punching power. This cylindrical bag is constructed of either top-grain leather, heavy canvas, or vinyl. The interior of the bag is generally filled with some type of cotton fiber. Heavy bags can weigh anywhere from 35 to 200 pounds, depending on the manufacturer. However, the average bag weighs approximately 85 pounds. Here are some points to keep in mind when training on the heavy bag:

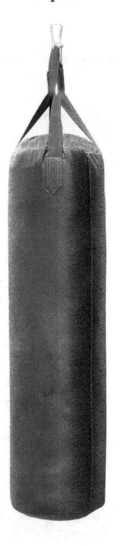

• Stay balanced. When delivering punishing blows on the bag, keep balanced. Maintain proper striking form and don't overextend your body.

• Be mobile. Avoid the tendency to remain stationary when working out on the heavy bag. Move around and vary the speed and direction of your footwork.

• Stay relaxed. Avoid tensing your muscles when striking the bag. Tensing your muscles will slow you down significantly.

• Throw combinations. As I mentioned earlier, avoid delivering one strike at a time. Learn to harmoniously integrate your kicks, punches, and strikes into devastating compound attacks.

• Keep your wrists straight. If your wrist bends or collapses on impact, you will either sprain or break it.

Q: Should I use hand wraps when working out on the heavy bag?

A: That's entirely up to you. Hand wraps can give your hands and wrists an added measure of protection when hitting a heavy bag. They provide support to the entire hand and wrist area and help prevent arthritis in later years. Hand wraps are along strips of cotton measuring 2 inches by 9 feet long that can be purchased at most sporting goods stores. If you do decide to use hand wraps in your training, be certain you learn how to wrap your hands correctly. (For information about specific hand-wrapping techniques, see *Heavy Bag Training: For Boxing, Mixed Martial Arts and Self-Defense.*)

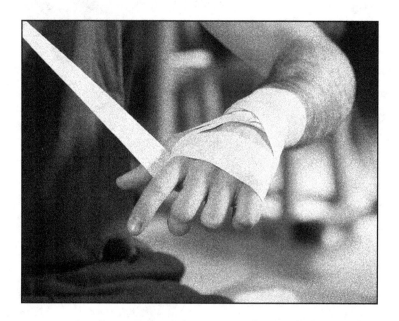

Q: Does the size or weight of the heavy bag matter?

A: Absolutely. The only way to develop the striking power necessary to floor a monstrous adversary is to train on a very heavy bag. There are numerous heavy bags on the market. For example, Ringside Equipment Company makes an excellent water bag that weighs 200 pounds and can withstand the most punishing blows. If you are looking to develop incredible knockout power, do not train on anything less than 75 pounds.

The Double-End Bag

The double-end bag is a small leather ball that is suspended from the ceiling and anchored to the floor with bungee cord. This training bag moves erratically and helps develop timing, accuracy, eye-hand coordination, footwork, defensive skills, and striking speed.

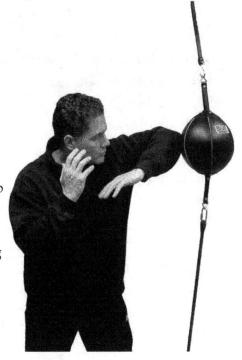

To use the double-end bag correctly, you must first make certain it is hung at a realistic height (approximately head level). This will allow you to effectively deploy your offensive arsenal. Defensive skills (parrying and slipping movements) can also be developed when the bag springs back at your face. Here are a few guidelines to follow when working out on the double-end bag.

• Don't lower your hands, even though it is a normal tendency. Be cognizant of your hand positioning at all times.

• Strike the bag solidly. If you don't hit the bag just right, it will bounce around uncontrollably. To control the movement of the bag, you must strike it solidly every time.

• Move your head around. When striking the bag, get into the habit of moving your head around arbitrarily. This will reinforce evasive skills.

• Be mobile. Avoid the tendency to just stand still and hit the bag. Strategic footwork should be included in your workout.

• Compound your strikes. Make it a habit to deliver combinations on the double-end bag. While this is not an easy task, it can be accomplished through consistent training.

The Body Opponent Bag

The body opponent bag (also called BOB) is a self-standing lifelike punching bag that's ideal when learning how to fight a bigger and heavier opponent.

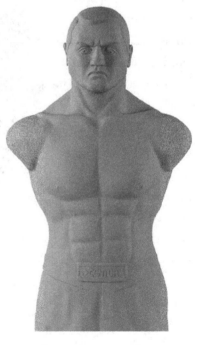

The base of the body opponent bag is constructed of hollow, hard plastic that allows you to adjust and increase the height of mannequin. This is an especially important feature when learning how to strike a significantly taller opponent. Also, when the base of the body opponent bag is completely filled, it will weigh approximately 270 pounds.

As you can imagine, a wide variety of kicks, punches, and strikes can be developed and ultimately perfected on the bag. However, the primary purpose of the BOB is to develop target accuracy for the following techniques:

• Head butt strikes

- All punching techniques

- Elbow and knee strikes

- Choking techniques

- Raking, clawing and gouging techniques

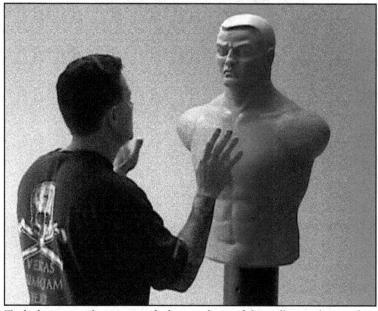

The body opponent bag is a great for learning how to fight a taller assailant. In this photo, the author prepares to strike his 7 foot opponent.

The Focus Mitts

The focus mitts are exceptional for developing accuracy, speed, target recognition, target selection, target impact, and timing in all offensive techniques. By placing the mitts at various angles and levels you can perform every conceivable kick, punch, or strike in your arsenal.

The Bigger They Are, The Harder They Fall

The focus mitt is constructed of durable leather and is designed to withstand tremendous punishment. Your training partner (called the feeder) plays a vital role in focus mitt workouts by controlling the tools you execute and the cadence of delivery. Here are a few guidelines for training on the focus mitts:

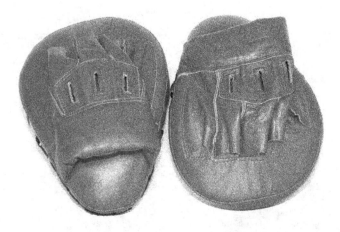

• Train with an experienced feeder. The intensity of your workout will depend largely upon the feeder's ability to effectively manipulate the mitts. Try to work with a feeder who knows how to safely push you to your physical limits.

• Don't slam the mitts into his blow. When holding the mitts, avoid slamming them into your partner's oncoming strike. This will negate the effectiveness of his blow and possibly injure his wrist or hand.

• Provide a reasonable amount of resistance with the mitts. This can be accomplished by tensing your hands and arms as the blow hits the surface of the mitt.

• Attack with the mitts. Don't forget that the feeder can also attack with various kicking techniques during the course of the workout. For example, swing at your partner from various angles to help him refine blocking and parrying movements.

The Striking Shield

The striking shield develops power in most of your kicks, punches, and strikes. This rectangular-shaped shield is constructed of foam and vinyl and is designed to withstand tremendous punishment. Your training partner plays a vital role in a good kicking-shield workout because he must hold the shield at the proper height and angle while simultaneously moving in and out of the ranges of combat. Here are some pointers for working on the striking shield:

• Brace yourself. When holding the striking shield, make concerted efforts to brace yourself for the impact of the kick or strike. Bend your knees, widen your stance, and plant your feet into the ground for greater stability.

• It's not just for kicking techniques. You can also deploy various knee and elbow strikes, punches, and head butts.

• Marry the shield to your body. Avoid the tendency to hold the shield away from your body. Make it a habit to keep the shield pressed closely against you. This will reduce the impact of the strike when it hits your body.

• Throw combinations on the shield. While the striking shield is excellent for "single tool" proficiency training, it can also be used for developing compound attack skills. Be creative and deliver logical combinations on the striking shield.

• Don't forget proper form. While the striking shield is primarily used for developing power, do not forget about proper form. Be certain to apply the correct body mechanics every time.

The Kicking Cylinder

The kicking cylinder is used for developing the hook kick and various knee strikes. This piece of equipment is approximately 4 feet high and is constructed of durable vinyl that can take a tremendous amount of abuse. When working out with your training partner, be certain that he braces himself for the impact.

Q: What is the benefit of shadow fighting?

A: Shadow fighting is the creative deployment of offensive and defensive tools and maneuvers against imaginary opponents. It requires intense mental concentration, honest self-analysis, and a deep commitment to improve yourself. One of the biggest mistakes during a shadow-fighting session is to simply "go through the motions." Remember to pay attention to the task at hand and your fighting skills will improve dramatically.

Shadow fighting is inexpensive—all you need is a full-length mirror and a place to work out. Proper shadow fighting develops speed, power, balance, footwork, compound attack skills, sound form, fluidity, and finesse. It even promotes a better understanding of the ranges of unarmed combat. Remember that you can never do too much shadow fighting. Here are some important points to keep in mind when shadow fighting:

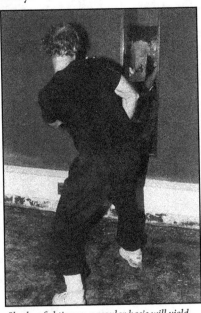

Shadow fighting on a regular basis will yield significant results when training.

• Be creative in your workout. Use your imagination and visualize realistic scenarios during your shadow-fighting routine. Imagine different types of opponents at various ranges of unarmed combat.

• Don't forget your defensive skills. Too many practitioners forget to incorporate defensive skills and techniques during their shadow-fighting workouts. Remember to include blocks, parries, slipping maneuvers, and evasive footwork.

• Keep it intense. Shadow fighting is not just a warm-up exercise. Do not make the mistake of simply going through the motions. If you want to reap the benefits, make certain that every shadow-fighting session is intense as well as challenging.

• Attack in combinations. One of the greatest mistakes you can make during a shadow-fighting workout is to throw one strike at a time. Get into the habit of attacking your imaginary opponent in strategic combinations using your kicks, punches, open-hand strikes, elbows, knees, etc. Remember that single-weapon victories are rare.

• Do not end with defense. When shadow fighting, avoid the tendency to end your compound attack with a defensive movement. This means that your imaginary adversary is still at large.

Q: I know that many professional boxers use the speed bag for training. Should I use it too?

A: No. The speed bag is a terrible training tool that develops bad habits for street combat. Working with the bag exposes your centerline, develops mechanical and unrealistic striking rhythms, and promotes improper body mechanics.   When it comes to reality-based self-defense training, stick with a heavy bag and body opponent bag.

Q: Can you recommend any other forms of training to better my odds against a larger opponent?

A: Yes. There are other forms of ancillary training that you can do to enhance your combative repertoire. Stick and knife fighting is a good start. Such types of weapons training will develop ambidexterity and eye-hand coordination, as well as offensive and defensive reaction time. Moreover, training with sticks and knives will also familiarize you with their strengths and weaknesses should they be used against you in a fight.

Q: Are there any training procedures that will help me defeat a massive adversary ?

A: There are three training methodologies (proficiency, conditioning, and street training) that should be integrated with your equipment-training program. All three methods are critical to defeating a larger and stronger adversary and they all can be performed on training equipment. Let us look at each method.

Training Methods

Training Methodology #1: Proficiency Training

Proficiency training is designed to sharpen one particular tool, technique, tactic, or maneuver at a time by executing it over and over again for a prescribed number of repetitions.

Proficiency training is often used to develop and sharpen the first-strike tools you will launch against your massive adversary. For example, one exercise might have you delivering finger jabs on the body opponent bag for 200 repetitions (with proper form and at various speeds). Techniques can even be practiced with the eyes closed to develop a kinesthetic "feel" for the movement. Remember to take your time with each repetition.

Here are three proficiency training routines (beginner, intermediate, and advanced) structured around the primary offensive tools that you will use against a stronger and larger adversary.

Beginner Level Proficiency Training Routine

Cadence: Pause 3 seconds between repetitions.

Offensive Technique	Repetitions
Finger jab	50
Web-hand strike	50
Lead hook punch	50
Lead shovel hook punch	50
Rear shovel hook punch	50
Lead uppercut punch	50
Rear uppercut punch	50

Intermediate Level Proficiency Training Routine

Cadence: Pause 1 second between repetitions.

Offensive Techniques	Repetitions
Finger jab	100
Web-hand strike	100
Lead hook punch	100
Lead shovel hook punch	100
Rear shovel hook punch	100
Lead uppercut punch	100
Rear uppercut punch	100

Advanced Level Proficiency Training Routine

Cadence: No pause between repetitions.

Offensive Techniques	Repetitions
Finger jab	150-200
Web-hand strike	150-200
Lead hook punch	150-200
Lead shovel hook punch	150-200
Rear shovel hook punch	150-200
Lead uppercut punch	150-200
Rear uppercut punch	150-200

Training Methodology #2: Conditioning Training

Conditioning training is designed to sharpen a fighter's arsenal while at the same time conditioning his entire body for combat. Moreover, it develops rhythm, balance, speed, agility, and footwork. This method of training should be practiced in a controlled environment, such as the studio, basement, or garage, to allow sufficient room for you and your training partner to really move around.

Conditioning training is primarily used to develop the secondary-strike tools that will be aimed at your adversary. Conditioning training requires you to execute your kicks, punches, and strikes in different combinations for 3- or 4-minute rounds. Once the round is over, rest for 30 seconds and then go again. A good workout consists of four to five rounds. Remember, your goal is to develop and sharpen your compound attack skills, so remember to maintain a proper breathing pattern; under no circumstances should you hold your breath. Here is a detailed list of all the offensive and defensive tools that should be incorporated into your conditioning training routine.

Offensive Techniques

Kicking range techniques: vertical kick, push kick, side kick, hook kick, shuffle side kick, and shuffle push kick.

Punching range techniques: finger jab, lead palm heel, rear palm heel, lead straight, rear cross, lead corkscrew punch, rear corkscrew punch, web-hand strike, lead horizontal hammer fist, rear horizontal hammer fist, horizontal knife hand, lead hook, rear hook, lead uppercut, rear uppercut, lead shovel hook, rear shovel hook, and rear vertical hammer fist (long arc).

Grappling range techniques (in the vertical plane): rear vertical knee, rear diagonal knee, rear vertical hammer fist (short arc), double thumb gouge, eye rake (vertical and horizontal), lead horizontal elbow, rear horizontal elbow, lead diagonal elbow (upward and downward), rear diagonal elbow (upward and downward), lead vertical elbow (upward and backward), rear vertical elbow (upward and backward), head butt (four directions), and foot stomp (forward and backward).

Defensive Tools and Maneuvers

Blocks: lead high block, rear high block, lead mid block, rear mid block, lead low block, rear low block, lead elbow block, rear elbow block, lead leg block, and rear leg block.

Parries: lead horizontal parry, rear horizontal parry, lead vertical parry, rear vertical parry, and rear catch.

Slipping: slipping right, slipping left, and snap back.

Evasive footwork: sidestep right, sidestep left, circle right, circle left, and retreat.

Training Methodology #3: Street Training

The last training methodology is called street training. This is the final preparation for the real thing. Since a typical physical confrontation (under ideal conditions) lasts approximately 20 to 30 seconds, you must prepare for this type of scenario.

Street training requires you to deliver your first strike and then follow up with explosive and powerful compound attacks for 20 to 30 seconds, resting for 1 minute, and then repeating the process. In the street-training methodology, it is essential to attack with 100-percent determination and give it everything you have.

Street training prepares you for the stress and fatigue of a real fight. It also develops speed, power, explosiveness, target selection, timing, footwork, and even balance. For example, stand in front of a heavy bag and deliver a quick push kick (this is your first-strike tool), then follow up with vicious compound attacks for 25 seconds (remember to keep the pressure on). Rest for 1 minute and then go again. It may sound easy to some, but I assure you that it is not. Here are just two versions of the street-training methodology.

The Gauntlet Drill

The gauntlet drill is a unique version of the street-training methodology. To perform this exercise you will need a minimum of 10 people, each holding one focus mitt. Divide the 10 people into two equal rows and make certain they hold the focus mitts at approximately head level.

Next, have the designated striker start from the top of the rows. From a fighting stance, have him deliver a lead straight/rear cross combination (also known as a one-two) as he moves steadily through the two rows. Once he works his way through the "gauntlet," he should quickly return to the starting position (top of the row) and begin again. You can also sharpen your defensive skills by having one or two people swing at you as you pass through the rows. Be careful!

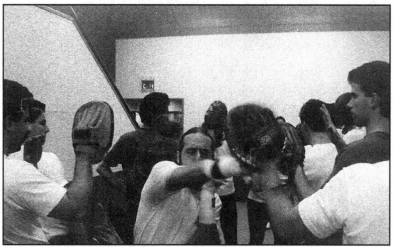

Here, one of my students perform the strenuous gauntlet drill. Notice how close the feeders are to the striker.

The Head-Hunter Drill

The head-hunter drill is another spin-off from the street-training methodology. This exercise is designed to sharpen and develop your hook punches. To perform this drill, assume a fighting stance and square off in front of a heavy bag or focus mitts. Then execute a lead and rear hook combination (back and forth) with maximum power and speed for 30 seconds. Do not stop executing your strikes until the time has elapsed. Rest for approximately 1 minute and then go again for three rounds. Be forewarned! This drill is exhausting.

The Bigger They Are, The Harder They Fall

Q: What is the greatest mistake people make when training?

A: Many practitioners are perfectionists and will habitually "freeze up" and berate themselves when they screw up during a training drill. This type of response can be disastrous in a real fight. Never let a mistake break your concentration or disrupt the fluidity of your movements.

Q: What about sparring?

A: Sparring is another important aspect of training that should not be neglected. Besides developing the many attributes of unarmed combat (timing, distancing, accuracy, compound attack skills, etc.) it will also condition your body. In addition, full contact sparring will allow you to experience what it feels like to be hit. While no one likes being hit, knowing how it feels will significantly reduce the shock that can occur from a real blow.

Moreover, sparring on a regular basis will help minimize some of the fear associated with combat, and this can be a strong confidence builder. Full-contact sparring will also help you learn just how effective a particular technique actually can be. Here are a few suggestions that will help you when sparring with a partner:

• Remember that it's not the real thing. While certain forms of sparring can be beneficial, never forget that they do not accurately represent the real danger and volatile dynamics of a vicious street fight.

• Occasionally wear different types of clothing when sparring. This is known as "attire training" and it will teach you a lot about the limitations of clothing when fighting.

• If you want to benefit from your sparring session, you will need to invest in a good pair of boxing gloves. The best gloves for full-contact sparring are ones that provide protection, comfort, and durability.

• Develop a strong hand guard. If you hold your hands up passively, you run the risk of being hit by your own boxing gloves when the opponent punches at your guard. Your arms must have a modicum of tension or your hand guard will lose its structural integrity.

• Do not panic. When you are hit during sparring, stay in control and do not panic. Remember to keep your hand guard up, keep moving, and look for the opportunity to counter your opponent. Too many practitioners "freak out" when hit and that is when the trouble really starts.

• Mix the ranges up. Avoid the tendency to spar and fight in only one range of unarmed combat. If you want your training to be realistic, strive to integrate the kicking, punching, and grappling ranges.

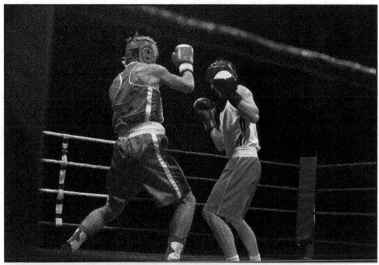

While certain forms of sparring can be beneficial, never forget that they do not accurately represent the real danger and volatile dynamics of a vicious street fight.

The Bigger They Are, The Harder They Fall

Q: Is there any particular style of sparring you recommend for training?

A: Since your goal is to be prepared to fight a larger and stronger adversary, it is best to spar with very large opponents—the bigger, the better. Moreover, when sparring, you want to employ the "blitz and disengage" method.

The "blitz and disengage" methodology closely resembles an actual street fight. The objective is to stay in the neutral zone until the opponent presents an opening. Once the window of opportunity presents itself, quickly move in and shower your adversary with a series of calculated blows and strikes. Remember to exploit your opponent's reaction dynamics. Once the assault is complete, disengage and relocate to safety.

Q: Are there any other full contact exercises that will prepare me for fighting a powerful opponent?

A: Hip fusing is an excellent full-contact drill that teaches you to stand your ground and overcome the fear of exchanging blows with a stronger opponent. This exercise is performed by connecting two fighters to each other with a 3-foot chain, which forces them to stay in punching range. The chain prevents the smaller practitioner from disengaging the punching range and literally "fuses" him to his massive enemy. This is especially beneficial for smaller fighters who habitually "hit and run" when sparring.

To perform the hip-fusing drill you will need the following items: boxing gloves, mouthpieces, headgear, two durable leather weight-lifting belts, a 3-foot chain, and two 7/16" snap links. Using the snap links, connect the chain to the belts and secure the belts to the fighters. The length of the chain may vary depending on the arm spans of the fighters. Depending on your level of conditioning, the hip-fusing drill can last anywhere from 30 seconds to 5 minutes. Remember that this drill should be performed with an opponent of greater size and strength.

Q: Can you give me a sample routine for cardio and equipment training?

A: Sure. Here is a typical training regimen:

Mon	Tues	Wed	Thurs	Fri	Sat
Focus Mitts	Run	Body Opponent Bag	Jumping Rope	Sparring	Sprint-ing
Heavy Bag		Double End Bag		Heavy Bag	
Kicking Cylinder		Shadow Fighting		Focus Mitts	

If your schedule or lifestyle permits you to perform more than three cardiovascular sessions per week, then by all means, do so. Ancillary training (stick and knife fighting, etc.) can also be added at your discretion.

The Bigger They Are, The Harder They Fall

Chapter Four
Armageddon

"The paradox of courage is that a man must be a little careless of his life even in order to keep it." - *G. K. Chesterton*

In the previous chapters you became familiar with both the strategic concepts and the physical training necessary to defeat an imposing adversary. Now it's time to see all of the principles put into action. In this chapter, I have provided you with 12 fighting scenarios demonstrating the knowledge, skills, and attitude necessary to beat a larger and more powerful adversary. Keep in mind that my opponent is significantly taller and has a 100-pound weight advantage over me.

In addition, since every self-defense confrontation is unique, these scenarios serve only as examples of the possible combinations that you can deploy in a fight. Finally, when reviewing the photographs, pay close attention to how I exploit my opponent's reaction dynamics.

Fighting Scenario #1

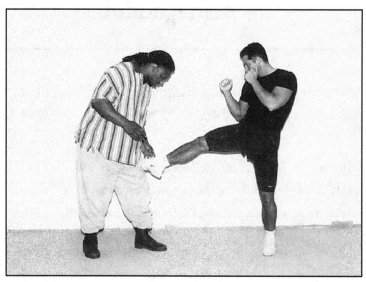

Step 1: From the neutral zone, Sammy Franco moves in with a quick push kick.

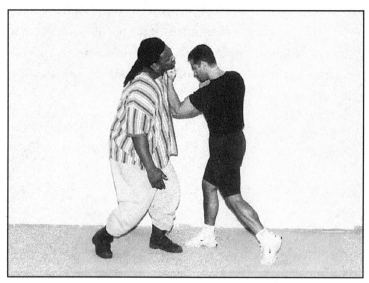

Step 2: Franco exploits his opponent's reaction dynamics with a rear uppercut punch.

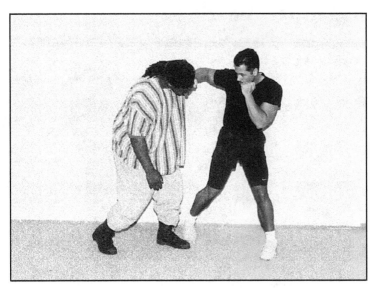

Step 3: Franco immediately follows with a lead hook punch.

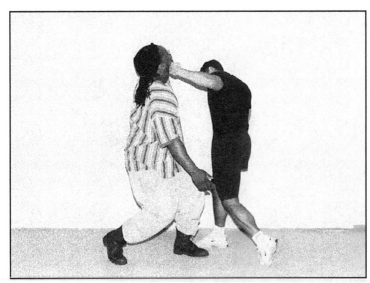

Step 4: The opponent is finished off with the rear hook.

Fighting Scenario #2

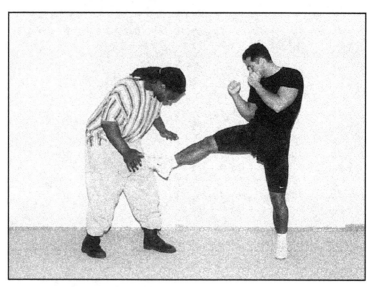

Step 1: From the neutral zone, the author moves in with a push kick to the opponent's thigh.

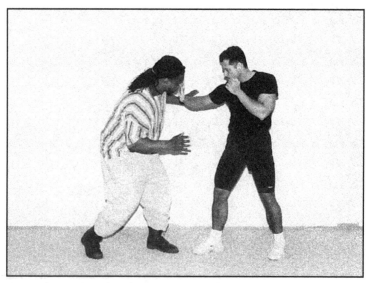

Step 2: The opponent drops his hands down and Franco attacks with the finger jab strike to his eyes.

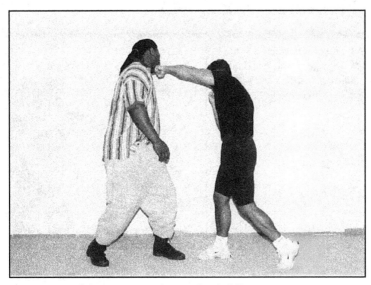

Step 3: A powerful rear cross punch immediately follows.

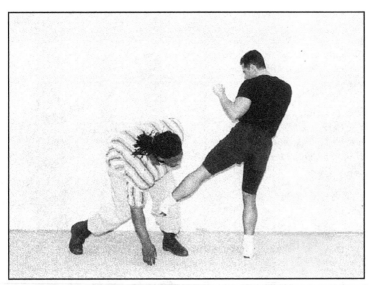

Step 4: The compound attack is completed with a hook kick to the opponent's knee.

Fighting Scenario #3

Step 1: Franco is threatened at the punching range of unarmed combat. He immediately strikes first with a finger jab to his opponents eyes.

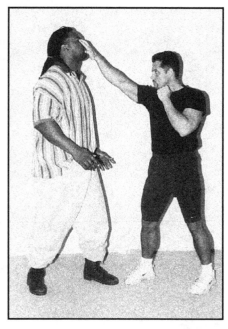

Step 2: Franco sees the window of opportunity and attacks with a rear web hand strike to the opponents throat.

Warning: the throat is considered a deadly force target and should only be attacked in situations that legally warrant the application of lethal force.

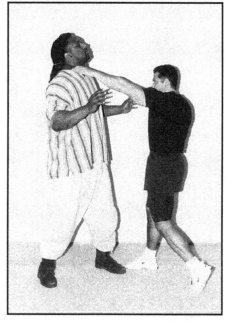

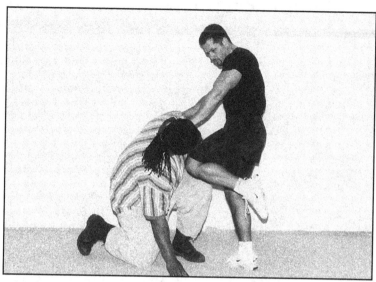

Step 3: The compound attack is completed with a rear vertical knee strike.

Important!

Once you have reviewed and studied all of the fighting scenarios, go back to the beginning of this chapter and visualize yourself in each scenario applying the exact techniques that I've employed against my opponent. Be certain that your mental images are crystal clear.

Fighting Scenario #4

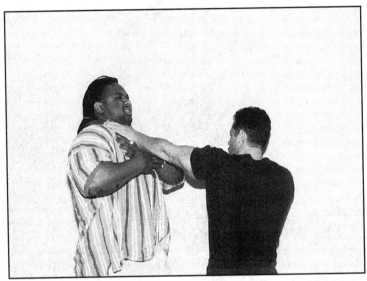

Step 1: From the punching range, the author attacks with the brutal web hand strike to the throat.

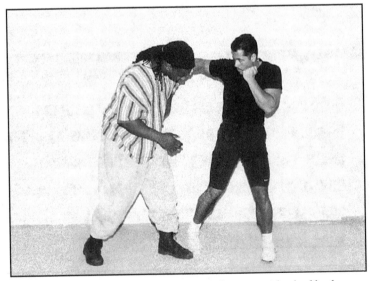

Step 2: Franco exploits his opponent's reaction dynamics with a lead hook punch.

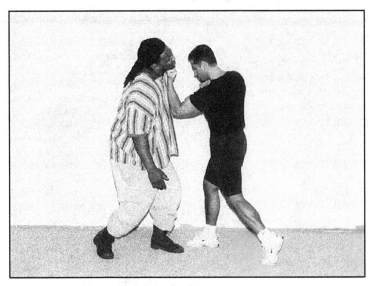

Step 3: Next, is the rear uppercut to the chin.

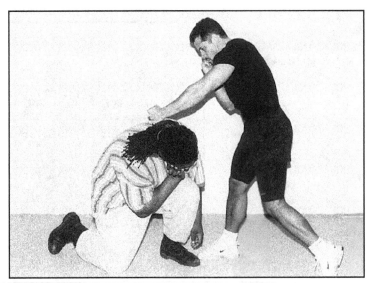

Step 4: The compound attack is finished with a rear hammer fist strike to the spine.

Fighting Scenario #5

Step 1: In this compound attack scenario, the author faces a 300 pound adversary in grappling range. Before his assailant can attack, Franco delivers a rear horizontal elbow strike to the solar plexus.

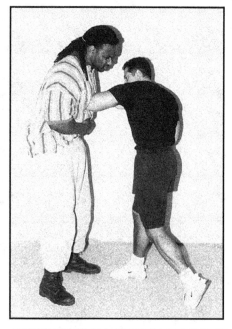

Step 2: The adversary falls backward and Franco maintains the offense flow with the lead hook punch to the head.

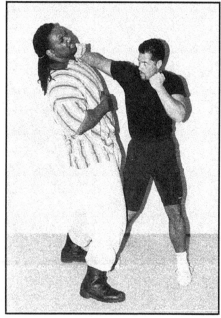

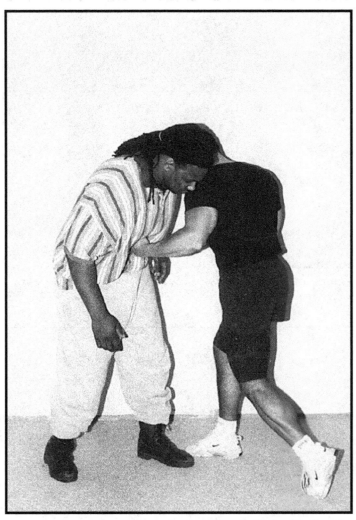

Step 3: The compound attack is completed with a powerful shovel book to the solar plexus.

Fighting Scenario #6

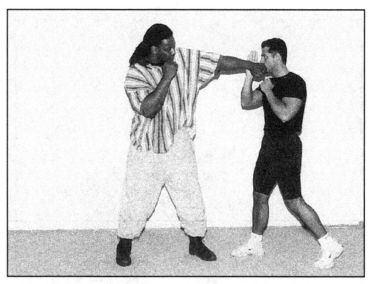

Step 1: The opponent attacks with a quick jab; Franco deflects the blow with a horizontal parry.

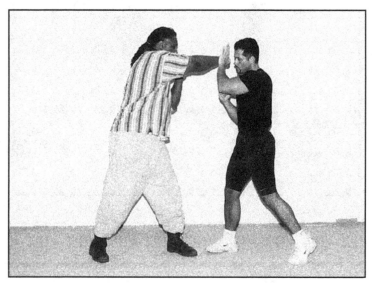

Step 2: The opponent follows up with the rear cross and Franco defends with the rear parry.

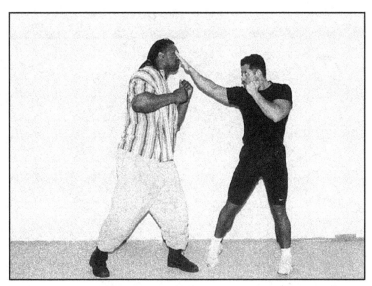

Step 3: Franco interrupts the opponent's offense flow by countering with a finger jab strike.

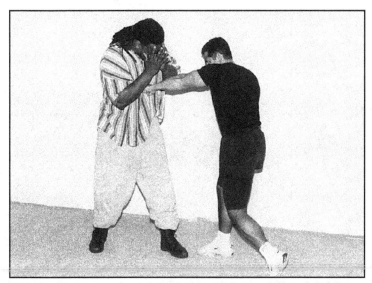

Step 4: Franco then drives a rear cross into his opponent's body.

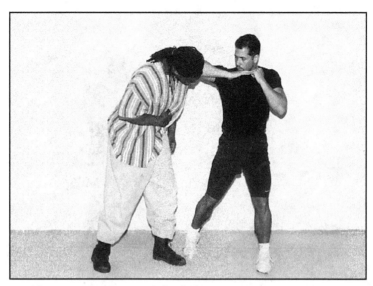

Step 5: Next, is a lead horizontal elbow strike.

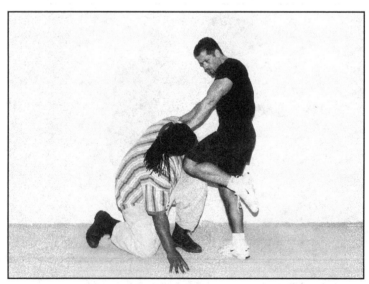

Step 6: The adversary is finished off with a rear vertical knee strike.

Fighting Scenario #7

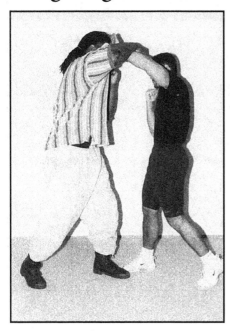

Step 1: In this scenario, Franco's adversary attempts to get the upper hand by attacking with an overhead punch. Franco immediately reacts with a rear high block.

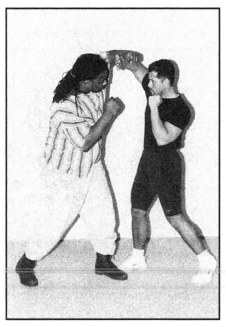

Step 2: The opponent attacks with another overhead punch.

Step 3: Franco disrupts his opponent's offensive flow and immediately counters with a rear horizontal elbow strike.

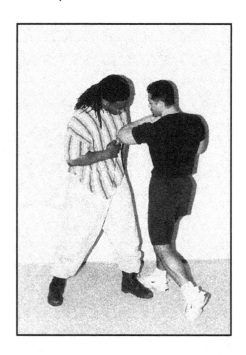

Step 4: Franco immediately follows up with a rear vertical knee strike.

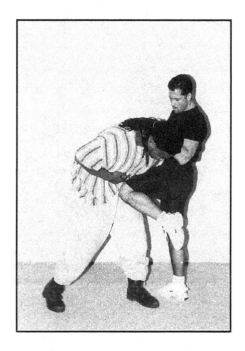

Fighting Scenario #8

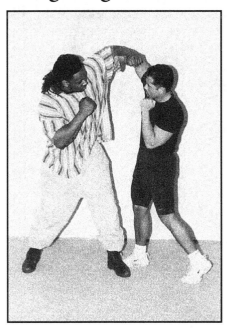

Step 1: Here, Franco is attacked and defends with a high block.

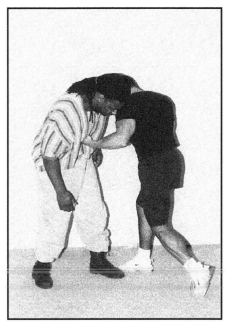

Step 2: Franco counters with a rear shovel punch.

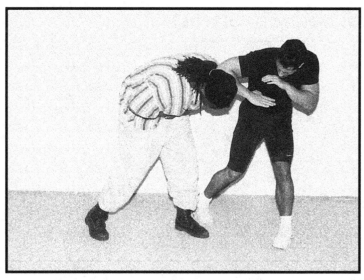

Step 3: He then follows with a lead diagonal elbow strike.

Step 4: Franco finishes the fight with a rear vertical knee strike to the face.

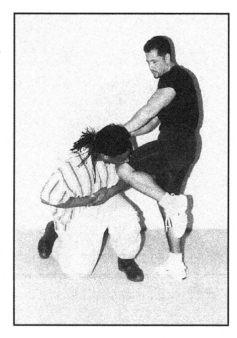

Fighting Scenario #9

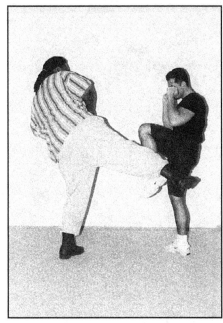

Step 1: The opponent attacks with a hook kick.

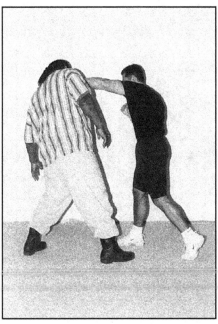

Step 2: Franco counters with a rear cross punch.

Step 3: He follows up with a lead uppercut punch to the assailant's chin.

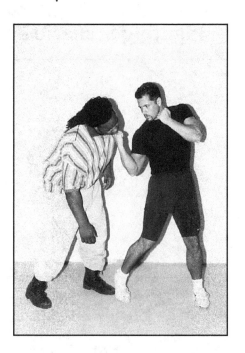

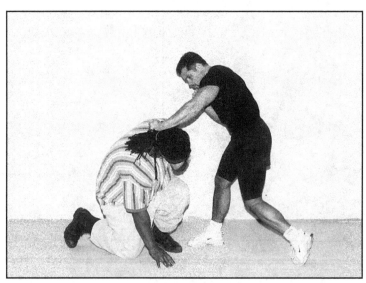

Step 4: Franco completes his compound attack with a hammer fist strike.

Fighting Scenario #10

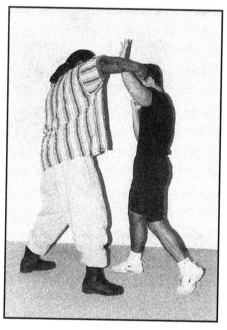

Step 1: The opponent attacks with a powerful haymaker. Franco uses a mid block to stop the assault.

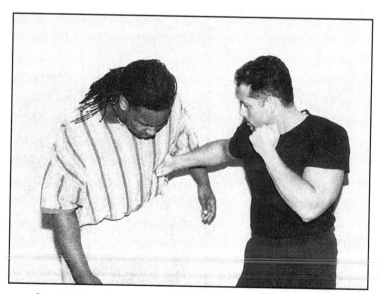

Step 2: Franco then counters with a right hook to the assailant's torso.

The Bigger They Are, The Harder They Fall

Step 3: He follows up with a rear uppercut punch.

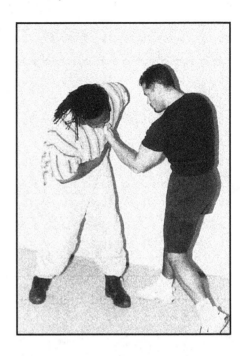

Step 4: A lead horizontal elbow is next.

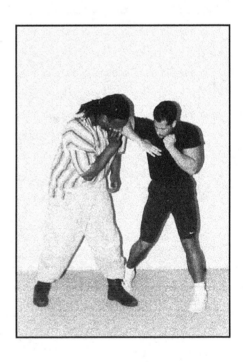

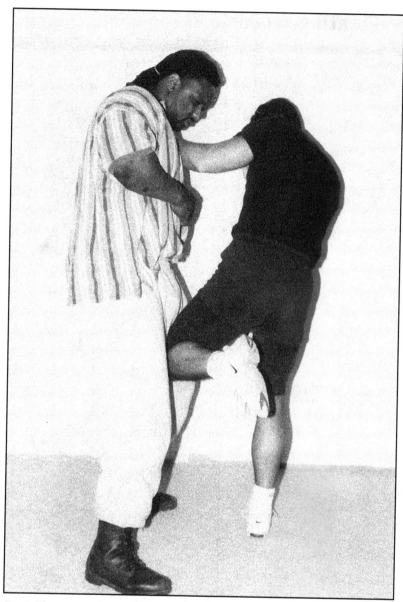

Step 5: The compound attack ends with a rear diagonal knee strike.

Fighting Scenario #11

Step 1: *The opponent attacks with an uppercut. Franco protects his body with a rear elbow block.*

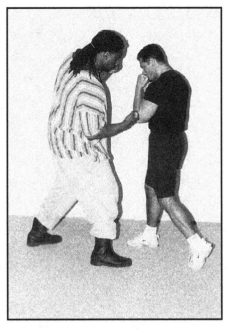

Step 2: *The defender maintains the range and immediately counters with a lead uppercut to the chin.*

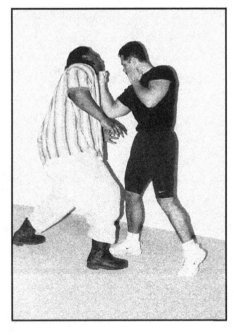

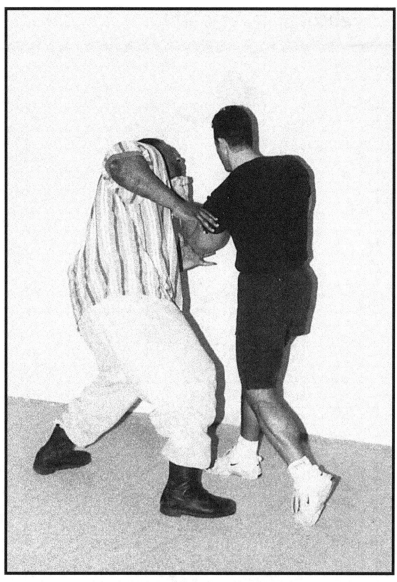

Step 3: Franco ends the fight with another powerful uppercut to the chin.

Fighting Scenario #12

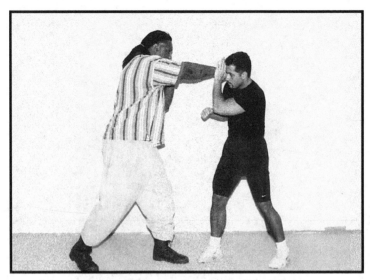

Step 1: The opponent gets the drop on Franco and attacks with the rear cross punch. Franco immediately deflects the blow.

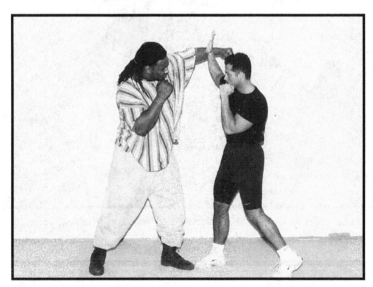

Step 2: The opponent follows up with a hook punch and Franco executes a mid block.

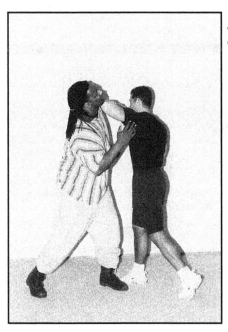

Step 3: Franco counters with a quick elbow strike to the chin.

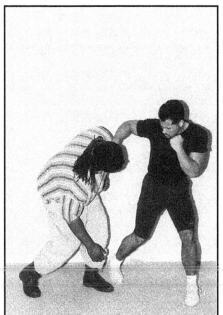

Step 4: He then follows up with a powerful hook punch.

The Bigger They Are, The Harder They Fall

Chapter Five
Grappling and Ground Fighting

"He that wrestles with us strengthens our nerves and sharpens our skill. Our antagonist is our helper."

- Edmund Burke (1729 - 1797)

Because of his superior size and strength, a larger man is more inclined to take you to the ground. In fact, the majority of self-defense confrontations will usually end up on the ground. To make matters even worse, a bigger and stronger person has a significant advantage in a ground fight. Therefore, in this chapter, I will talk about the many important issues surrounding grappling and ground fighting a larger and stronger man.

Q: I'm really good with my hands and feet - why do I have to know how to grapple and ground fight?

A: Regardless of how proficient you may be with your striking arsenal, there is a good chance that the fight will still go to the ground. You must also remember that a larger and stronger opponent may instinctively try to rush and tackle you or otherwise smother you with his body. The bottom line is, if your adversary is determined to take you to the ground, he will most likely succeed. Therefore, it's critical that you have the knowledge and skills necessary to handle close-quarter grappling and ground fighting.

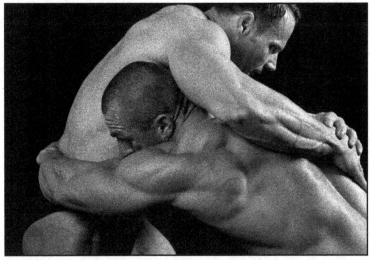

Big guys love to grapple, especially with smaller people.

Q: What can happen if I am not prepared for the ground fight?

A: If you're not prepared to fight in grappling range (vertical and horizontal planes), then you may be subjected to premature exhaustion, panic, severe injury, asphyxiation, possible death, absolute humiliation, and inevitable defeat.

Q: Okay, okay I get your point. So what do I need to know?

A: You must be able to fight in both the vertical and horizontal grappling planes. The vertical grappling range refers to when you are standing toe-to-toe with the opponent, and horizontal grappling range is when you are ground fighting.

Q: I heard from a top Brazilian grappler that the best chance to win a fight against a bigger and stronger opponent is to close the distance and take him to the ground. Do you agree?

A: Absolutely not! While I do believe that you should be prepared for the possibility of a ground fight, I do not believe that you should try to initiate one. Always try to fight him while you are standing on both of your feet. Remember, mobility is a vital component to your survival. Once you go to the ground with your opponent, mobility and movement is gone.

Q: Why don't you advocate taking a bigger opponent to the ground?

A: There are just too many risks and dangers when ground fighting in a street fight. For example, since ground fighting requires maximal body entanglement, it is virtually impossible to defend against multiple attackers (you never know if your opponent has friends close by).

Moreover, it's extremely difficult to defend against knives and other edged weapons when grappling with your assailant on the floor. Who's to say that your massive opponent is not concealing a knife in his pocket? Even the most seasoned grappler will openly admit that ground fighting can be exhausting and time consuming. And time is one thing that you don't have much of in a street fight.

Furthermore, ground fighting also requires that you be acutely aware of the terrain. For example, broken glass, sharp metal, or broken wood littering the ground can be extremely dangerous. Finally, the opponent's sheer size will pose a serious problem for you. If he is exceptionally large, he can simply smother you with his weight and mass.

Q: Is there any situation or circumstance that would ever justify taking a larger and stronger opponent to the ground?

A: I can only think of one - if you are losing a range of combat. If, for example, your opponent is beating the hell out of you in punching range and it's impossible for you to disengage, you have no other choice but to close the range, take him to the ground, establish a strategic position, and hopefully choke him out.

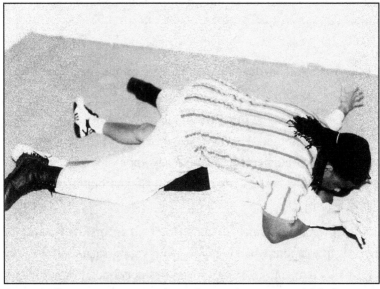

Beware! A larger opponent can easily smother you during a ground fight. Be especially careful when fighting in this range of unarmed combat.

Q: What is the most common takedown a larger opponent will attempt?

A: That really depends on your opponents skill level. For example, if he's a knowledgeable mixed martial artist he might try to bring you down using either a single or double leg takedown. However, if he's your run-of-the-mill street thug, he'll most likely use a body tackle known as a "bums rush" - haphazardly rushing forward and plowing his body into yours.

Q: How do I defend against a body tackle?

A: One of the best methods of defending against a charge (i.e., a body tackle) is through contact evasion. Contact evasion involves physically moving (sidestepping) or manipulating your body to avoid being tackled by your opponent.

The key to a successful contact evasion is proper timing—you should always wait until the very last moment. Move too soon and your assailant will follow you. If you move too late, he will maul you.

Another effective technique is called a stiff arm jam. The stiff-arm jam is a very effective method of negating the destructive force of both the upper and mid body tackles.

To perform the technique, simultaneously lower your base (height change to level of entry) and extend both of your arms forward. Both of your palms should make contact with the assailant's upper chest and shoulder. Be certain to pull your fingers back to avoid accidental sprains or breaks. Your objective is to instantaneously negate or "jam" the overwhelming force of the takedown.

If the adversary attempts the upper body tackle, the palms of your hands should make contact on both sides of his chest region. If he attempts a mid body tackle, lower your base and have your palms jam him at his shoulders. One more thing, it's critical that you remember to change your height to match your assailant's level of entry.

Q: What about moving backward against a body tackle?

A: Don't do it! The adversary will only generate greater momentum and inevitably take you down to the floor. Again, moving laterally is your safest bet or using the stiff-arm jam technique.

Q: Are there any other types of takedown that I should be concerned about?

A: The double-leg takedown is one that skilled grapplers are more inclined to use.

Q: Should I use contact evasion against a double-leg takedown?

A: Yes, and if there's not enough time to move sideways you can also sprawl. Actually, sprawling is one of the best methods of countering an assailant who attempts either a single- or double-leg takedown. Sprawling is accomplished by lowering your hips to the ground while simultaneously shooting both of your legs back. The primary objective of sprawling is to get your legs back and force your body weight onto your assailant's shoulders and head.

Q: Can I sprawl against an upper body tackle?

A: Since the opponent doesn't significantly lower his torso for an upper body tackle, it's very difficult to apply the sprawling technique.

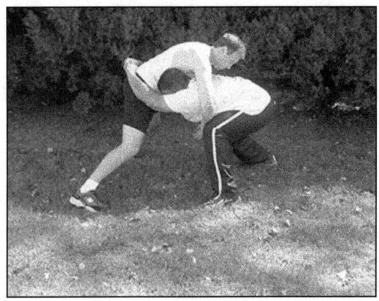

STEP 1: In this photo, the man on the right attempts a mid body tackle. The self-defense practitioner (left) immediately sprawls his legs back and drops his hips into the grappler's head and shoulders.

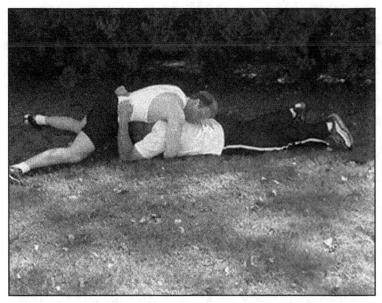

STEP 2: *The defender (left) maintains steady pressure, which drives his opponent straight to the ground.*

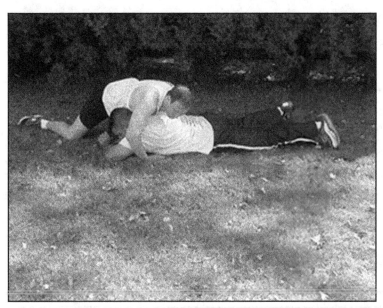

STEP 3: *The defender (top) quickly pivots and rotates his body around the opponent's back.*

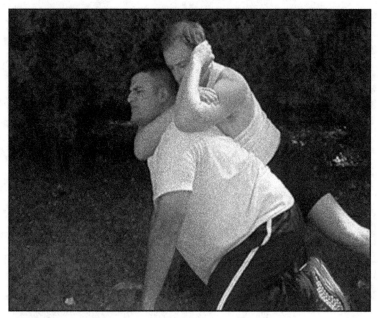

STEP 4: *The man on top executes a modified neck choke.*

Q: Are there any drills that can help me defend against a body tackle?

A: Yes. There is the sidestepping drill that refines evasion skills and enhances your sense of timing. To practice the drill, begin by assuming a stance (such as fighting, de-escalation, natural, or knife defense) and have your training partner stand approximately 10 feet from you. Next, without telegraphing his intentions, your training partner should charge at you full-speed. If you're standing in a left (orthodox) stance, quickly step to the left with your left foot and have your right leg follow an equal distance. Your partner should pass you and you should be balanced and ready to effectively counterattack. Remember to practice the sidestepping drill with different stances, at various distances (8 and 6 feet), in different lighting conditions, and while standing on different surfaces.

Q: What is the best way of getting out of my assailant's leg guard?

A: To answer this question, you must first know exactly what the guard position is. The guard, also known as the scissors hold, is a defensive ground-fighting position in which the opponent wraps both of his legs around your waist. This position is a favorite among many jiu-jitsu fighters and grapplers since it allows them to trap their opponents and apply various submission techniques.

Escaping from the assailant's leg guard is not an easy task, but there are two effective methods. First is the striking method, in which you attack the assailant with a flurry of powerful hammer-fist blows to the groin region until the scissors hold is released, or shower his face with a barrage of punches. Just be on the lookout for any possible arm bars or triangle chokes that he may attempt when you attack his head and face. The second method of escaping the guard is the submission hold method, in which you strategically twist and torque the assailant's ankle and knee.

Q: What is my most important objective when ground fighting my opponent?

A: Simple, get up from the ground as quickly as possible.

Q: Why should I avoid applying control and restraint techniques when fighting a larger adversary?

A: While control and restraint techniques (submission holds) are a necessary component of your combat cache, they do possess inherent risks and limitations. Control and restraint techniques will not work effectively against large and flexible assailants. Also, if your opponent is high on some drug like PCP, you can forget it. Most importantly, your opponent's size and strength can often negate the effectiveness of many submission techniques.

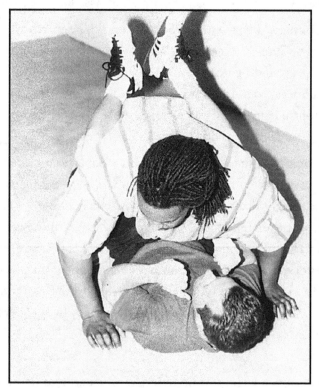

Ground fighting someone of greater size is very difficult. It's often impossible to apply certain submission holds on a massive opponent. In this photo, the man on the bottom cannot wrap his leg guard around his enormous opponent.

Q: If I must ground fight a larger adversary can I use "nuclear tactics"?

A: In CFA, nuclear tactics refer to specific techniques designed to inflict immediate and irreversible damage rendering the enemy helpless. The only time you can use nuclear ground-fighting tactics is when you are faced with a life-and-death encounter where lethal force is warranted and justified in the eyes of the law, such as against criminal assault with intent to kill.

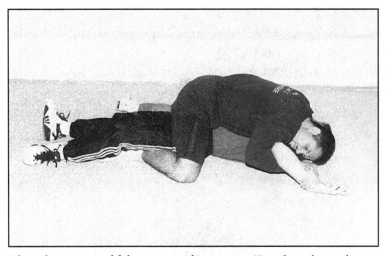

It's much easier ground fighting a man of average size. Here, the author applies a submission hold. Notice how an opponent of reasonable size makes Franco's submission technique look effortless.

Nuclear Tactics for Street Fighting

- **Biting**
- **Tearing**
- **Crushing**
- **Choking techniques**
- **Gouging and raking techniques**

Q: So, exactly what is my strategy if my opponent attempts to take me to the ground?

A: First, stay mobile (use contact evasion) by moving on the balls of your feet. Second, strike first and try to create as much damage to the opponent as you can before he locks up with you. Remember, never kick at a charging attacker, as this will throw you off balance, allowing your assailant to control the takedown. Fourth, when your assailant locks up with you, sprawl or embrace him and attack with a variety of close-quarter tools. Fifth, when the fight goes to the ground, immediately go for the mounted position and try to maintain it. Sixth, once the mounted position is established, attack the assailant with a barrage of vicious strikes to his facial targets until he is neutralized. If deadly force is warranted, immediately apply nuclear ground-fighting techniques.

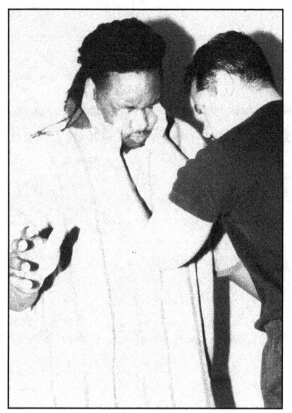

Don't forget that nuclear tactics can also be applied when standing toe to toe with your adversary. Here, Franco attacks his opponent with a double thumb gouge in the grappling range.

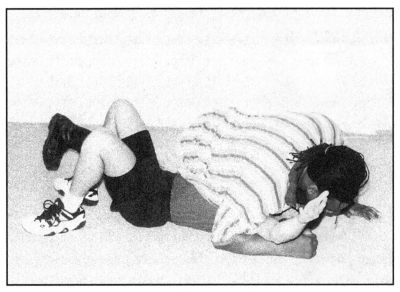

Positional asphyxia is one of your biggest concerns when ground fighting a larger and heavier opponent. Here, the man on the bottom is in serious trouble!

Q: What is my biggest concern when ground fighting a larger adversary?

A: Positional asphyxia, which is the arrangement, placement, or positioning of your opponent's body so that it interrupts your breathing and causes unconsciousness or possibly death.

Q: How do I prevent positional asphyxia?

A: It's really simple: don't let your opponent establish the top mounted position or any other position that will otherwise smother your face or compress your lungs. If and when your fight goes to the ground, it is critical that you immediately try to acquire the mounted position or any other strategic placement that will prevent your adversary from using his size and weight to impair your breathing.

The Bigger They Are, The Harder They Fall

Q: But what if my opponent takes me to the ground and gets the mounted position?

A: There are many escape techniques that can be applied when an opponent has mounted you. However, since this book deals with fighting a massive adversary of extreme weight, you must realize that escape techniques and maneuvers will not work, no matter how skilled you are in the grappling arts. It's a sad but true fact. The bottom line is that physics are physics and at some point there is nothing you can do.

Imagine a professional football player—let's say an extremely massive front lineman—mounted on top of you with all of his weight dropped on your chest. In terms of maneuvering and strategic positioning, there is very little that you can do at this point. (This is assuming that you are significantly smaller and lighter than your mounted adversary.) In such a situation, your only hope is that the opponent may lower his head close enough to yours so that you can either bite into his face (nose, ears, and the throat) or forcefully drive your thumbs into his eyes. Your objective is to create intense pain so he wants to get off you.

Q: I heard that the only way to beat an opponent who knows jiu-jitsu is to study jiu-jitsu. Is that true?

A: No, it's not. Keep in mind that there are more than 50 different grappling or wrestling arts out there today. To say that jiu-jitsu is superior to other grappling arts is absurd. However, one thing is certain: if you are a one dimensional fighter who practices only one style of martial arts (karate, kung-fu, aikido, judo, etc.), you will get killed in a street fight. To defeat a massive adversary who possesses grappling skills (such as a practitioner of jiu-jitsu), you must be multidimensional in your training. You must be a hybrid fighter who possesses a variety of combat skills (kicking, punching, grappling, weapons training, etc.). The day of the 1-dimensional fighter is gone forever!

Q: Are there any other aspects of ground fighting that I should be aware of?

A: Ground-fighting positions are very important. There are four general positions that you will find yourself in when grappling with a larger and stronger adversary. They are:

Mounted position: This is when you are sitting on top of your assailant's torso or chest.

Perpendicular mount position: This is when both your legs are on one side of your assailant's body, and your body runs perpendicular to your assailant's.

Chest to back position: This is when your chest is on the assailant's back (it does not matter if you are on top of him, he is on top of you, or you are both on your sides).

Opposite pole position: This is when both you and your assailant are facing opposite directions (this often occurs when sprawling against your adversary).

Q: What about the guard position?

A: While the guard position (when you wrap your legs around your assailant's torso) is a critical position when ground fighting someone of reasonable size, it has severe limitations when applied on a massive opponent. Nevertheless, if you can wrap your legs around your hulking adversary, then do so; but if you can't, you'd better try one of the other ground-fighting positions.

Q: Is there anything else I should be aware of when ground fighting a larger and stronger adversary?

The Bigger They Are, The Harder They Fall

A: Yes. Under no circumstances should you ever roll over onto your stomach. This is perilous for several reasons, including that the opponent can easily choke you out and deliver a barrage of blows to your head, neck, and back while it is virtually impossible for you to defend yourself.

Q: What if my opponent grabs me when I am standing?

A: Grab defenses are simple to learn. Actually, any person who attempts a grab is a real amateur in the world of self-defense. He is clearly uneducated and is setting himself up for a vicious counterattack, regardless of his size.

Typically, you have three possible options when assaulted with a grab, choke, or hold from a standing position. I have created a unique, use-of-force response system called "MAP," which stands for moderate, aggressive, and passive responses.

M: In a moderate response, you counter your opponent with a control/restraint submission hold.

A: If you decide on an aggressive response, you counter your enemy with destructive and conclusive counterblows.

P: Answering with a passive response has you nullifying the assault without injuring your adversary.

However, when assaulted by a larger and stronger adversary, it is important to always counter with an aggressive response. This will maximize your safety and end the altercation quickly. The following photographs will illustrate a few scenarios employing the aggressive response method.

Defense against a one-hand wrist grab

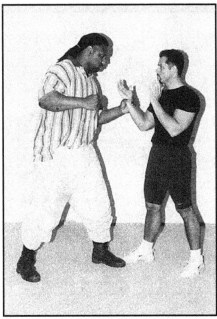

Step 1: In this photo, the opponent grabs Franco's right hand. Franco slowly raises his left hand to protect himself and set up his counterstrike.

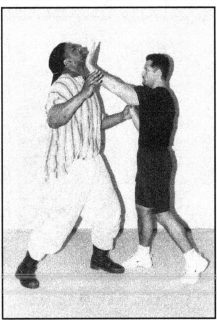

Step 2: Franco immediately counters with a rear palm heel strike to his opponent's chin

Defense against a two-hand wrist grab

Step 1: Franco attempts to de-escalate his hostile adversary. The opponent ignores Franco and grabs both of his wrists.

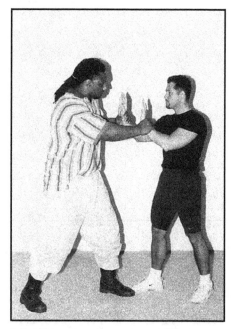

Step 2: To escape the grab, Franco raises his left hand up and over his right hand and forcefully pulls it back.

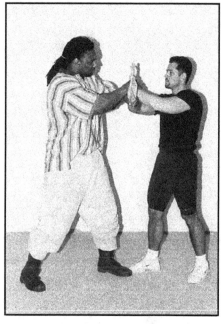

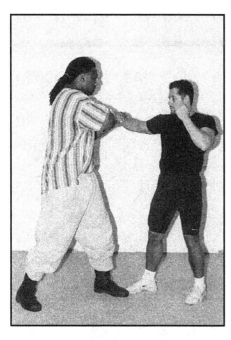

Step 3: Once his left hand is free, he grabs his opponents wrist.

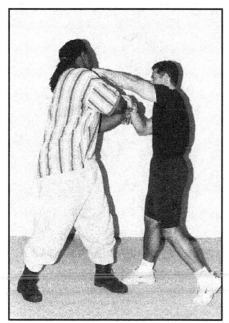

Step 4: Franco counters with the rear cross to the face.

Defense against a two-hand wrist grab (low)

Step 1: The opponent grabs both of Franco's wrists.

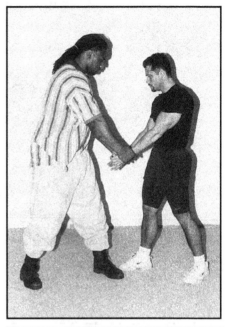

Step 2: To escape from the grab, Franco places his right hand over his opponents wrist.

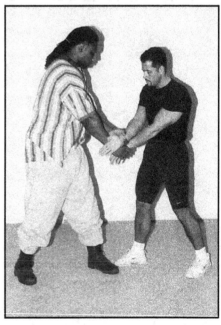

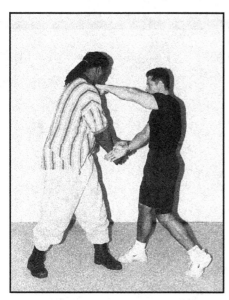

Step 3: Franco pulls his left hand out and counters with the rear cross punch.

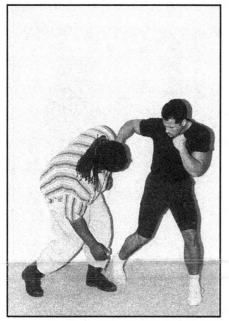

Step 4: Franco follows up with a lead hook punch to the head.

Defense against a shoulder grab

Step 1: The assailant grabs Franco's right shoulder.

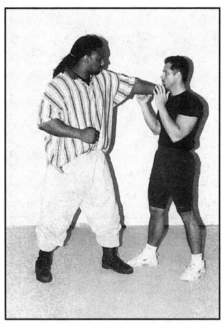

Step 2: Franco instantly traps his opponent's hand and counters with a web hand strike to the opponent's throat.

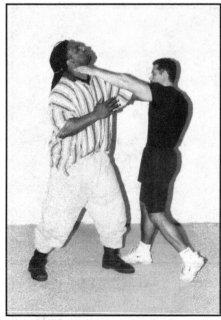

Defense against a two-hand throat choke

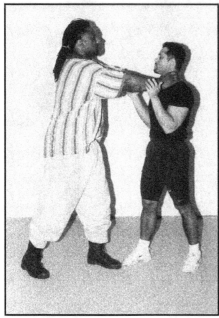

Step 1: The opponent rushes forward and chokes Franco with two hands.

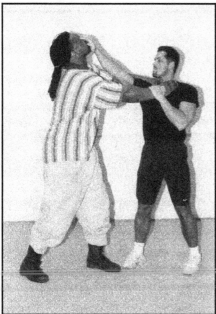

Step 2: Franco pulls down his opponents hand and simultaneously counters with a forceful finger jab strike to the eyes.

Step 3: He follows with a web-hand strike to the throat.

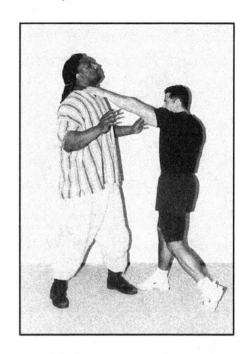

Step 4: Franco completes his counter attack with a lead uppercut strike to the opponent's chin.

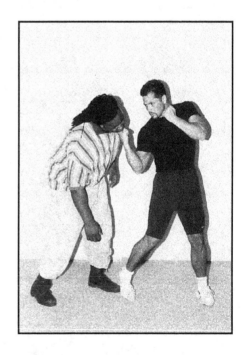

Defense against a two-hand throat choke (rear)

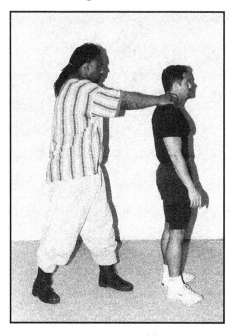

Step 1: The adversary grabs Franco by the throat.

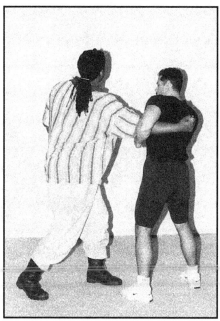

Step 2: Here Franco steps forward with his right leg and simultaneously swings his left arm around his opponent's elbow.

The Bigger They Are, The Harder They Fall

Step 3: Once Franco secures his opponent's arm, he counters with a web hand strike to the throat.

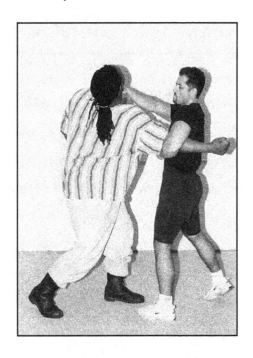

Step 4: Franco follows up with an elbow strike.

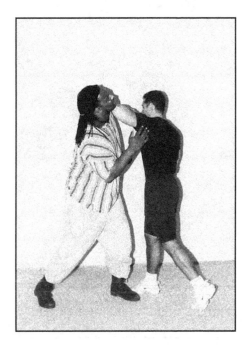

Defense against a side head lock

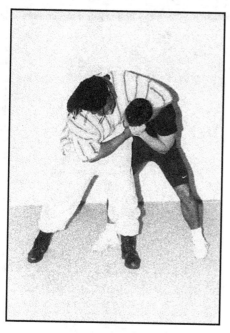

Step 1: The assailant places Franco and a headlock. Franco immediately widens his stance and simultaneously turns his head into the opponents side (this action helps prevent him from losing oxygen).

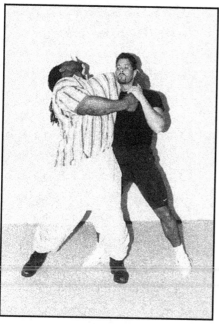

Step 2: Franco then reaches over his opponent's back and places his middle finger under the assailants nose (septum region) and forces the massive man backwards.

169

The Bigger They Are, The Harder They Fall

Step 3: Franco then attacks by crushing his opponents windpipe with his left hand. Warning! Attacking the throat should only be used in life and death self-defense situations that warrant the use of deadly force.

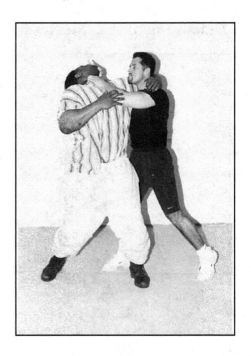

Glossary

The following terms are defined in the context of Contemporary Fighting Arts and its related concepts. In many instances, the definitions bear little resemblance to those found in a standard dictionary.

A

accuracy—The precise or exact projection of force. Accuracy is also defined as the ability to execute a combative movement with precision and exactness.

adaptability—The ability to physically and psychologically adjust to new or different conditions or circumstances of combat.

advanced first-strike tools—Offensive techniques that are specifically used when confronted with multiple opponents.

aerobic exercise—Literally, "with air." Exercise that elevates the heart rate to a training level for a prolonged period of time, usually 30 minutes.

affective preparedness – One of the three components of preparedness. Affective preparedness means being emotionally, philosophically, and spiritually prepared for the strains of combat. See cognitive preparedness and psychomotor preparedness.

aggression—Hostile and injurious behavior directed toward a person.

aggressive response—One of the three possible counters when assaulted by a grab, choke, or hold from a standing position. Aggressive response requires you to counter the enemy with destructive blows and strikes. See moderate response and passive response.

aggressive hand positioning—Placement of hands so as to imply aggressive or hostile intentions.

agility—An attribute of combat. One's ability to move his or her body quickly and gracefully.

amalgamation—A scientific process of uniting or merging.

ambidextrous—The ability to perform with equal facility on both the right and left sides of the body.

anabolic steroids – synthetic chemical compounds that resemble the male sex hormone testosterone. This performance-enhancing drug is known to increase lean muscle mass, strength, and endurance.

analysis and integration—One of the five elements of CFA's mental component. This is the painstaking process of breaking down various elements, concepts, sciences, and disciplines into their atomic parts, and then methodically and strategically analyzing, experimenting, and drastically modifying the information so that it fulfills three combative requirements: efficiency, effectiveness, and safety. Only then is it finally integrated into the CFA system.

anatomical striking targets—The various anatomical body targets that can be struck and which are especially vulnerable to potential harm. They include: the eyes, temple, nose, chin, back of neck, front of neck, solar plexus, ribs, groin, thighs, knees, shins, and instep.

assailant—A person who threatens or attacks another person.

assault—The threat or willful attempt to inflict injury upon the person of another.

assault and battery—The unlawful touching of another person without justification.

assessment—The process of rapidly gathering, analyzing, and accurately evaluating information in terms of threat and danger. You can assess people, places, actions, and objects.

attack—Offensive action designed to physically control, injure, or kill another person.

attitude—One of the three factors that determine who wins a street fight. Attitude means being emotionally, philosophically, and spiritually liberated from societal and religious mores. See skills and knowledge.

attributes of combat—The physical, mental, and spiritual qualities that enhance combat skills and tactics.

awareness—Perception or knowledge of people, places, actions, and objects. (In CFA, there are three categories of tactical awareness: criminal awareness, situational awareness, and self-awareness.)

B

balance—One's ability to maintain equilibrium while stationary or moving.

blading the body—Strategically positioning your body at a 45-degree angle.

blitz and disengage—A style of sparring whereby a fighter moves into a range of combat, unleashes a strategic compound attack, and then quickly disengages to a safe distance. Of all sparring methodologies, the blitz and disengage most closely resembles a real street fight.

block—A defensive tool designed to intercept the assailant's attack by placing a non-vital target between the assailant's strike and your vital body target.

body composition—The ratio of fat to lean body tissue.

body language—Nonverbal communication through posture, gestures, and facial expressions.

body mechanics—Technically precise body movement during the execution of a body weapon, defensive technique, or other fighting maneuver.

body tackle – A tackle that occurs when your opponent haphazardly rushes forward and plows his body into yours.

body weapon—Also known as a tool, one of the various body parts that can be used to strike or otherwise injure or kill a criminal assailant.

burn out—A negative emotional state acquired by physically over- training. Some symptoms include: illness, boredom, anxiety, disinterest in training, and general sluggishness.

C

cadence—Coordinating tempo and rhythm to establish a timing pattern of movement.

cardiorespiratory conditioning—The component of physical fitness that deals with the heart, lungs, and circulatory system.

centerline—An imaginary vertical line that divides your body in half and which contains many of your vital anatomical targets.

choke holds—Holds that impair the flow of blood or oxygen to the brain.

circular movements—Movements that follow the direction of a curve.

close-quarter combat—One of the three ranges of knife and bludgeon combat. At this distance, you can strike, slash, or stab your assailant with a variety of close-quarter techniques.

cognitive development—One of the five elements of CFA's mental component. The process of developing and enhancing your fighting skills through specific mental exercises and techniques. See analysis and integration, killer instinct, philosophy, and strategic/tactical development.

cognitive exercises—Various mental exercises used to enhance fighting skills and tactics.

cognitive preparedness – One of the three components of preparedness. Cognitive preparedness means being equipped with the strategic concepts, principles, and general knowledge of combat. See affective preparedness and psychomotor preparedness.

combat-oriented training—Training that is specifically related to the harsh realities of both armed and unarmed combat. See ritual-oriented training and sport-oriented training.

combative arts—The various arts of war. See martial arts.

combative attributes—See attributes of combat.

combative fitness—A state characterized by cardiorespiratory and muscular/skeletal conditioning, as well as proper body composition.

combative mentality—Also known as the killer instinct, this is a combative state of mind necessary for fighting. See killer instinct.

combat ranges—The various ranges of unarmed combat.

combative utility—The quality of condition of being combatively useful.

combination(s)—See compound attack.

common peroneal nerve—A pressure point area located approximately four to six inches above the knee on the midline of the outside of the thigh.

composure—A combative attribute. Composure is a quiet and focused mind-set that enables you to acquire your combative agenda.

compound attack—One of the five conventional methods of attack. Two or more body weapons launched in strategic succession whereby the fighter overwhelms his assailant with a flurry of full speed, full-force blows.

conditioning training—A CFA training methodology requiring the practitioner to deliver a variety of offensive and defensive combinations for a 4-minute period. See proficiency training and street training.

contact evasion—Physically moving or manipulating your body to avoid being tackled by the adversary.

Contemporary Fighting Arts—A modern martial art and self-defense system made up of three parts: physical, mental, and spiritual.

conventional ground-fighting tools—Specific ground-fighting techniques designed to control, restrain, and temporarily incapacitate your adversary. Some conventional ground fighting tactics include: submission holds, locks, certain choking techniques, and specific striking techniques.

coordination—A physical attribute characterized by the ability to perform a technique or movement with efficiency, balance, and accuracy.

counterattack—Offensive action made to counter an assailant's initial attack.

courage—A combative attribute. The state of mind and spirit that enables a fighter to face danger and vicissitudes with confidence, resolution, and bravery.

creatine monohydrate—A tasteless and odorless white powder that mimics some of the effects of anabolic steroids. Creatine is a safe body-building product that can benefit anyone who wants to increase their strength, endurance, and lean muscle mass.

criminal awareness—One of the three categories of CFA awareness. It involves a general understanding and knowledge of the nature and dynamics of a criminal's motivations, mentalities, methods, and capabilities to perpetrate violent crime. See situational awareness and self-awareness.

criminal justice—The study of criminal law and the procedures associated with its enforcement.

criminology—The scientific study of crime and criminals.

cross-stepping—The process of crossing one foot in front of or behind the other when moving.

crushing tactics—Nuclear grappling-range techniques designed to crush the assailant's anatomical targets.

D

deadly force—Weapons or techniques that may result in unconsciousness, permanent disfigurement, or death.

deception—A combative attribute. A stratagem whereby you delude your assailant.

decisiveness—A combative attribute. The ability to follow a tactical course of action that is unwavering and focused.

defense—The ability to strategically thwart an assailant's attack (armed or unarmed).

defensive flow—A progression of continuous defensive responses.

defensive mentality—A defensive mind-set.

defensive reaction time—The elapsed time between an assailant's physical attack and your defensive response to that attack. See offensive reaction time.

demeanor—A person's outward behavior. One of the essential factors to consider when assessing a threatening individual.

diet—A lifestyle of healthy eating.

disingenuous vocalization—The strategic and deceptive utilization of words to successfully launch a preemptive strike at your adversary.

distancing—The ability to quickly understand spatial relationships and how they relate to combat.

distractionary tactics—Various verbal and physical tactics designed to distract your adversary.

double-end bag—A small leather ball hung from the ceiling and anchored to the floor with bungee cord. It helps develop striking accuracy, speed, timing, eye-hand coordination, footwork and overall defensive skills.

double-leg takedown—A takedown that occurs when your opponent shoots for both of your legs to force you to the ground.

E

ectomorph—One of the three somatotypes. A body type characterized by a high degree of slenderness, angularity, and fragility. See endomorph and mesomorph.

effectiveness—One of the three criteria for a CFA body weapon, technique, tactic, or maneuver. It means the ability to produce a desired effect. See efficiency and safety.

efficiency—One of the three criteria for a CFA body weapon, technique, tactic, or maneuver. It means the ability to reach an objective quickly and economically. See effectiveness and safety.

emotionless—A combative attribute. Being temporarily devoid of human feeling.

endomorph—One of the three somatotypes. A body type characterized by a high degree of roundness, softness, and body fat. See ectomorph and mesomorph.

evasion—A defensive maneuver that allows you to strategically maneuver your body away from the assailant's strike.

evasive sidestepping—Evasive footwork where the practitioner moves to either the right or left side.

evasiveness—A combative attribute. The ability to avoid threat or danger.

excessive force—An amount of force that exceeds the need for a particular event and is unjustified in the eyes of the law.

experimentation—The painstaking process of testing a combative hypothesis or theory.

explosiveness—A combative attribute that is characterized by a sudden outburst of violent energy.

F

fear—A strong and unpleasant emotion caused by the anticipation or awareness of threat or danger. There are three stages of fear in order of intensity: fright, panic, and terror. See fright, panic, and terror.

feeder—A skilled technician who manipulates the focus mitts.

femoral nerve—A pressure point area located approximately 6 inches above the knee on the inside of the thigh.

fighting stance—Any one of the stances used in CFA's system. A strategic posture you can assume when face-to-face with an unarmed assailant(s). The fighting stance is generally used after you have launched your first-strike tool.

fight-or-flight syndrome—A response of the sympathetic nervous system to a fearful and threatening situation, during which it prepares your body to either fight or flee from the perceived danger.

finesse—A combative attribute. The ability to skillfully execute a movement or a series of movements with grace and refinement.

first strike—Proactive force used to interrupt the initial stages of an assault before it becomes a self-defense situation.

first-strike principle—A CFA principle that states that when physical danger is imminent and you have no other tactical option but to fight back, you should strike first, strike fast, and strike with authority and keep the pressure on.

first-strike stance—One of the stances used in CFA's system. A strategic posture used prior to initiating a first strike.

first-strike tools—Specific offensive tools designed to initiate a preemptive strike against your adversary.

fisted blows – Hand blows delivered with a clenched fist.

five tactical options – The five strategic responses you can make in a self-defense situation, listed in order of increasing level of resistance: comply, escape, de-escalate, assert, and fight back.

flexibility—The muscles' ability to move through maximum natural ranges. See muscular/skeletal conditioning.

focus mitts—Durable leather hand mitts used to develop and sharpen offensive and defensive skills.

footwork—Quick, economical steps performed on the balls of the feet while you are relaxed, alert, and balanced. Footwork is structured around four general movements: forward, backward, right, and left.

fractal tool—Offensive or defensive tools that can be used in more than one combat range.

fright—The first stage of fear; quick and sudden fear. See panic and terror.

G

grappling range—One of the three ranges of unarmed combat. Grappling range is the closest distance of unarmed combat from which you can employ a wide variety of close-quarter tools and techniques. The grappling range of unarmed combat is also divided into two planes: vertical (standing) and horizontal (ground fighting). See kicking range and punching range.

grappling-range tools—The various body tools and techniques that are employed in the grappling range of unarmed combat, including head butts; biting, tearing, clawing, crushing, and gouging tactics; foot stomps, horizontal, vertical, and diagonal elbow strikes, vertical and diagonal knee strikes, chokes, strangles, joint locks, and holds. See punching range tools and kicking range tools.

ground fighting—Also known as the horizontal grappling plane, this is fighting that takes place on the ground.

guard—Also known as the hand guard, this refers to a fighter's hand positioning.

guard position—Also known as leg guard or scissors hold, this is a ground-fighting position in which a fighter is on his back holding his opponent between his legs.

H

hand positioning—See guard.

hand wraps—Long strips of cotton that are wrapped around the hands and wrists for greater protection.

haymaker—A wild and telegraphed swing of the arms executed by an unskilled fighter.

head-hunter—A fighter who primarily attacks the head.

heavy bag—A large cylindrical bag used to develop kicking, punching, or striking power.

high-line kick—One of the two different classifications of a kick. A kick that is directed to targets above an assailant's waist level. See low-line kick.

hip fusing—A full-contact drill that teaches a fighter to "stand his ground" and overcome the fear of exchanging blows with a stronger opponent. This exercise is performed by connecting two fighters with a 3-foot chain, forcing them to fight in the punching range of unarmed combat.

histrionics—The field of theatrics or acting.

hook kick—A circular kick that can be delivered in both kicking and punching ranges.

hook punch—A circular punch that can be delivered in both the punching and grappling ranges.

I

impact power—Destructive force generated by mass and velocity.

impact training—A training exercise that develops pain tolerance.

incapacitate—To disable an assailant by rendering him unconscious or damaging his bones, joints, or organs.

initiative—Making the first offensive move in combat.

inside position—The area between the opponent's arms, where he has the greatest amount of control.

intent—One of the essential factors to consider when assessing a threatening individual. The assailant's purpose or motive. See demeanor, positioning, range, and weapon capability.

intuition—The innate ability to know or sense something without the use of rational thought.

J

joint lock—A grappling-range technique that immobilizes the

assailant's joint.

K

kick—A sudden, forceful strike with the foot.

kicking range—One of the three ranges of unarmed combat. Kicking range is the furthest distance of unarmed combat wherein you use your legs to strike an assailant. See grappling range and punching range.

kicking-range tools—The various body weapons employed in the kicking range of unarmed combat, including side kicks, push kicks, hook kicks, and vertical kicks.

killer instinct—A cold, primal mentality that surges to your consciousness and turns you into a vicious fighter.

kinesics—The study of nonlinguistic body movement communications. (For example, eye movement, shrugs, or facial gestures.)

kinesiology—The study of principles and mechanics of human movement.

kinesthetic perception—The ability to accurately feel your body during the execution of a particular movement.

knowledge—One of the three factors that determine who will win a street fight. Knowledge means knowing and understanding how to fight. See skills and attitude.

L

lead side -The side of the body that faces an assailant.

leg guard—See guard position.

linear movement—Movements that follow the path of a straight line.

low-maintenance tool—Offensive and defensive tools that require the least amount of training and practice to maintain proficiency. Low maintenance tools generally do not require preliminary stretching.

low-line kick—One of the two different classifications of a kick. A kick that is directed to targets below the assailant's waist level. (See high-line kick.)

lock—See joint lock.

M

maneuver—To manipulate into a strategically desired position.

MAP—An acronym that stands for moderate, aggressive, passive. MAP provides the practitioner with three possible responses to various grabs, chokes, and holds that occur from a standing position. See aggressive response, moderate response, and passive response.

martial arts—The "arts of war."

masking—The process of concealing your true feelings from your opponent by manipulating and managing your body language.

mechanics—(See body mechanics.)

mental attributes—The various cognitive qualities that enhance your fighting skills.

mental component—One of the three vital components of the CFA system. The mental component includes the cerebral aspects of fighting including the killer instinct, strategic and tactical development, analysis and integration, philosophy, and cognitive development. See physical component and spiritual component.

mesomorph—One of the three somatotypes. A body type classified by a high degree of muscularity and strength. The mesomorph possesses the ideal physique for unarmed combat. See ectomorph and endomorph.

mobility—A combative attribute. The ability to move your body quickly and freely while balanced. See footwork.

moderate response—One of the three possible counters when assaulted by a grab, choke, or hold from a standing position. Moderate response requires you to counter your opponent with a control and restraint (submission hold). See aggressive response and passive response.

modern martial art—A pragmatic combat art that has evolved to meet the demands and characteristics of the present time.

mounted position—A dominant ground-fighting position where a fighter straddles his opponent.

muscular endurance—The muscles' ability to perform the same motion or task repeatedly for a prolonged period of time.

muscular flexibility—The muscles' ability to move through maximum natural ranges.

muscular strength—The maximum force that can be exerted by a particular muscle or muscle group against resistance.

muscular/skeletal conditioning—An element of physical fitness that entails muscular strength, endurance, and flexibility.

N

naked choke—A throat choke executed from the chest to back position. This secure choke is executed with two hands and it can be performed while standing, kneeling, and ground fighting with the opponent.

neutralize—See incapacitate.

neutral zone—The distance outside the kicking range at which neither the practitioner nor the assailant can touch the other.

nonaggressive physiology—Strategic body language used prior to initiating a first strike.

nontelegraphic movement—Body mechanics or movements that do not inform an assailant of your intentions.

nuclear ground-fighting tools—Specific grappling range tools designed to inflict immediate and irreversible damage. Nuclear tools and tactics include biting tactics, tearing tactics, crushing tactics, continuous choking tactics, gouging techniques, raking tactics, and all striking techniques.

O

offense—The armed and unarmed means and methods of attacking a criminal assailant.

offensive flow—Continuous offensive movements (kicks, blows, and strikes) with unbroken continuity that ultimately neutralize or terminate the opponent. See compound attack.

offensive reaction time—The elapsed time between target selection and target impaction.

one-mindedness—A state of deep concentration wherein you are free from all distractions (internal and external).

ostrich defense—One of the biggest mistakes one can make when defending against an opponent. This is when the practitioner looks away from that which he fears (punches, kicks, and strikes). His mentality is, "If I can't see it, it can't hurt me."

P

pain tolerance—Your ability to physically and psychologically withstand pain.

panic—The second stage of fear; overpowering fear. See fright and terror.

parry—A defensive technique: a quick, forceful slap that redirects an assailant's linear attack. There are two types of parries: horizontal and vertical.

passive response—One of the three possible counters when assaulted by a grab, choke, or hold from a standing position. Passive response requires you to nullify the assault without injuring your adversary. See aggressive response and moderate response.

patience—A combative attribute. The ability to endure and tolerate difficulty.

perception—Interpretation of vital information acquired from your senses when faced with a potentially threatening situation.

philosophical resolution—The act of analyzing and answering various questions concerning the use of violence in defense of yourself and others.

philosophy—One of the five aspects of CFA's mental component. A deep state of introspection whereby you methodically resolve critical questions concerning the use of force in defense of yourself or others.

physical attributes—The numerous physical qualities that enhance your combative skills and abilities.

physical component—One of the three vital components of the CFA system. The physical component includes the physical aspects of fighting, such as physical fitness, weapon/technique mastery, and combative attributes. See mental component and spiritual component.

physical conditioning—See combative fitness.

physical fitness—See combative fitness.

positional asphyxia—The arrangement, placement, or positioning of your opponent's body in such a way as to interrupt your breathing and cause unconsciousness or possibly death.

positioning—The spatial relationship of the assailant to the assailed person in terms of target exposure, escape, angle of attack, and various other strategic considerations.

post-traumatic syndrome—A group of symptoms that may occur in the aftermath of a violent confrontation with a criminal assailant. Common symptoms of post-traumatic syndrome include denial, shock, fear, anger, severe depression, sleeping and eating disorders, societal withdrawal, and paranoia.

power—A physical attribute of armed and unarmed combat. The amount of force you can generate when striking an anatomical target.

power generators—Specific points on your body that generate impact power. There are three anatomical power generators: shoulders, hips, and feet.

precision—See accuracy.

preemptive strike—See first strike.

premise—An axiom, concept, rule, or any other valid reason to modify or go beyond that which has been established.

preparedness—A state of being ready for combat. There are three components of preparedness: affective preparedness, cognitive preparedness, and psychomotor preparedness.

proficiency training—A CFA training methodology requiring the practitioner to execute a specific body weapon, technique, maneuver, or tactic over and over for a prescribed number of repetitions. See conditioning training and street training.

proxemics—The study of the nature and effect of man's personal space.

proximity—The ability to maintain a strategically safe distance from a threatening individual.

pseudospeciation—A combative attribute. The tendency to assign subhuman and inferior qualities to a threatening assailant.

psychological conditioning—The process of conditioning the mind for the horrors and rigors of real combat.

psychomotor preparedness—One of the three components of preparedness. Psychomotor preparedness means possessing all of the physical skills and attributes necessary to defeat a formidable adversary. See affective preparedness and cognitive preparedness.

punch—A quick, forceful strike of the fists.

punching range—One of the three ranges of unarmed combat. Punching range is the mid range of unarmed combat from which the fighter uses his hands to strike his assailant. See kicking range and grappling range.

punching-range tools—The various body weapons that are employed in the punching range of unarmed combat, including finger jabs, palm-heel strikes, rear cross, knife-hand strikes, horizontal and shovel hooks, uppercuts, and hammer-fist strikes. See grappling-range tools and kicking-range tools.

Q

qualities of combat—See attributes of combat.

R

range—The spatial relationship between a fighter and a threatening assailant.

range deficiency—The inability to effectively fight and defend in all ranges of combat (armed and unarmed).

range manipulation—A combative attribute. The strategic manipulation of combat ranges.

range proficiency—A combative attribute. The ability to effectively fight and defend in all ranges of combat (armed and unarmed).

ranges of engagement—See combat ranges.

ranges of unarmed combat—The three distances (kicking range, punching range, and grappling range) a fighter might physically engage with an assailant while involved in unarmed combat.

reaction dynamics—The assailant's physical response or reaction to a particular tool, technique, or weapon after initial contact is made.

reaction time—The elapsed time between a stimulus and the response to that particular stimulus. See offensive reaction time and defensive reaction time.

rear cross—A straight punch delivered from the rear hand that crosses from right to left (if in a left stance) or left to right (if in a right stance).

rear side—The side of the body furthest from the assailant. See lead side.

reasonable force—That degree of force which is not excessive for a particular event and which is appropriate in protecting yourself or others.

refinement—The strategic and methodical process of improving or perfecting.

relocation principle—Also known as relocating, this is a street-fighting tactic that requires you to immediately move to a new location (usually by flanking your adversary) after delivering a compound attack.

repetition—Performing a single movement, exercise, strike, or action continuously for a specific period.

research—A scientific investigation or inquiry.

rhythm—Movements characterized by the natural ebb and flow of related elements.

ritual-oriented training—Formalized training that is conducted without intrinsic purpose. See combat-oriented training and sport-oriented training.

S

safety—One of the three criteria for a CFA body weapon, technique, maneuver, or tactic. It means that the tool, technique, maneuver or tactic provides the least amount of danger and risk for the practitioner. See efficiency and effectiveness.

scissors hold—See guard position.

self-awareness—One of the three categories of CFA awareness. Knowing and understanding yourself. This includes aspects of yourself which may provoke criminal violence and which will promote a proper and strong reaction to an attack. See criminal awareness and situational awareness.

self-confidence—Having trust and faith in yourself.

self-enlightenment—The state of knowing your capabilities, limitations, character traits, feelings, general attributes, and motivations. See self-awareness.

set—A term used to describe a grouping of repetitions.

shadow fighting—A CFA training exercise used to develop and refine your tools, techniques, and attributes of armed and unarmed combat.

situational awareness—One of the three categories of CFA

awareness. A state of being totally alert to your immediate surroundings, including people, places, objects, and actions. (See criminal awareness and self-awareness.)

skeletal alignment—The proper alignment or arrangement of your body. Skeletal alignment maximizes the structural integrity of striking tools.

skills—One of the three factors that determine who will win a street fight. Skills refers to psychomotor proficiency with the tools and techniques of combat. See Attitude and Knowledge.

slipping—A defensive maneuver that permits you to avoid an assailant's linear blow without stepping out of range. Slipping can be accomplished by quickly snapping the head and upper torso sideways (right or left) to avoid the blow.

snap back—A defensive maneuver that permits you to avoid an assailant's linear and circular blows without stepping out of range. The snap back can be accomplished by quickly snapping the head backward to avoid the assailant's blow.

somatotypes—A method of classifying human body types or builds into three different categories: endomorph, mesomorph, and ectomorph. See endomorph, mesomorph, and ectomorph.

sparring—A training exercise where two or more fighters fight each other while wearing protective equipment.

speed—A physical attribute of armed and unarmed combat. The rate or a measure of the rapid rate of motion.

spiritual component—One of the three vital components of the CFA system. The spiritual component includes the metaphysical issues and aspects of existence. See physical component and mental component.

sport-oriented training—Training that is geared for competition and governed by a set of rules. See combat-oriented training and ritual-oriented training.

sprawling—A grappling technique used to counter a double- or single-leg takedown.

square off—To be face-to-face with a hostile or threatening assailant who is about to attack you.

stance—One of the many strategic postures you assume prior to or during armed or unarmed combat.

stick fighting—Fighting that takes place with either one or two sticks.

strategic positioning—Tactically positioning yourself to either escape, move behind a barrier, or use a makeshift weapon.

strategic/tactical development—One of the five elements of CFA's mental component.

strategy—A carefully planned method of achieving your goal of engaging an assailant under advantageous conditions.

street fight—A spontaneous and violent confrontation between two or more individuals wherein no rules apply.

street fighter—An unorthodox combatant who has no formal training. His combative skills and tactics are usually developed in the street by the process of trial and error.

street training—A CFA training methodology requiring the practitioner to deliver explosive compound attacks for 10 to 20 seconds. See condition ng training and proficiency training.

strength training—The process of developing muscular strength through systematic application of progressive resistance.

striking art—A combat art that relies predominantly on striking techniques to neutralize or terminate a criminal attacker.

striking shield—A rectangular shield constructed of foam and vinyl used to develop power in your kicks, punches, and strikes.

striking tool—A natural body weapon that impacts with the assailant's anatomical target.

strong side—The strongest and most coordinated side of your body.

structure—A definite and organized pattern.

style—The distinct manner in which a fighter executes or performs his combat skills.

stylistic integration—The purposeful and scientific collection of tools and techniques from various disciplines, which are strategically integrated and dramatically altered to meet three essential criteria: efficiency, effectiveness, and combative safety.

submission holds—Also known as control and restraint techniques, many of these locks and holds create sufficient pain to cause the adversary to submit.

system—The unification of principles, philosophies, rules, strategies, methodologies, tools, and techniques of a particular method of combat.

T

tactic—The skill of using the available means to achieve an end.

target awareness—A combative attribute that encompasses five strategic principles: target orientation, target recognition, target selection, target impaction, and target exploitation.

target exploitation—A combative attribute. The strategic maximization of your assailant's reaction dynamics during a fight. Target exploitation can be applied in both armed and unarmed encounters.

target impaction—The successful striking of the appropriate anatomical target.

target orientation—A combative attribute. Having a workable knowledge of the assailant's anatomical targets.

target recognition—The ability to immediately recognize appropriate anatomical targets during an emergency self-defense situation.

target selection—The process of mentally selecting the appropriate anatomical target for your self-defense situation. This is predicated on certain factors, including proper force response, assailant's positioning, and range.

target stare—A form of telegraphing in which you stare at the anatomical target you intend to strike.

target zones—The three areas in which an assailant's anatomical targets are located. (See zone one, zone two and zone three.)

technique—A systematic procedure by which a task is accomplished.

telegraphic cognizance—A combative attribute. The ability to recognize both verbal and non-verbal signs of aggression or assault.

telegraphing—Unintentionally making your intentions known to your adversary.

tempo—The speed or rate at which you speak.

terminate—To kill.

terror—The third stage of fear; defined as overpowering fear. See fright and panic.

timing—A physical and mental attribute of armed and unarmed combat. Your ability to execute a movement at the optimum moment.

tone—The overall quality or character of your voice.

tool—See body weapon.

traditional martial arts—Any martial art that fails to evolve and change to meet the demands and characteristics of its present environment.

traditional style/system—See traditional martial arts.

training drills—The various exercises and drills aimed at perfecting combat skills, attributes, and tactics.

U

unified mind—A mind free and clear of distractions and focused on the combative situation.

use of force response—A combative attribute. Selecting the appropriate level of force for a particular emergency self-defense situation.

V

viciousness—A combative attribute. The propensity to be extremely violent and destructive often characterized by intense savagery.

violence—The intentional utilization of physical force to coerce, injure, cripple, or kill.

visualization—Also known as mental visualization or mental imagery. The purposeful formation of mental images and scenarios in the mind's eye.

W

warm-up—A series of mild exercises, stretches, and movements designed to prepare you for more intense exercise.

weak side—The weaker and more uncoordinated side of your body.

weapon and technique mastery—A component of CFA's physical component. The kinesthetic and psychomotor development of a weapon or combative technique.

weapon capability—An assailant's ability to use and attack with a particular weapon.

Y

yell—A loud and aggressive scream or shout used for various strategic reasons.

Z

zone one—Anatomical targets related to your senses, including the eyes, temple, nose, chin, and back of neck.

zone three—Anatomical targets related to your mobility, including thighs, knees, shins, and instep.

zone two—Anatomical targets related to your breathing, including front of neck, solar plexus, ribs, and groin.

The Bigger They Are, The Harder They Fall

About The Author

With over 30 years of experience, Sammy Franco is one of the world's foremost authorities on armed and unarmed self-defense. Highly regarded as a leading innovator in combat sciences, Mr. Franco was one of the premier pioneers in the field of "reality-based" self-defense and martial arts instruction.

Sammy Franco is perhaps best known as the founder and creator of Contemporary Fighting Arts (CFA), a state-of-the-art offensive-based combat system that is specifically designed for real-world self-defense. CFA is a sophisticated and practical system of self-defense, designed specifically to provide efficient and effective methods to avoid, defuse, confront, and neutralize both armed and unarmed attackers.

CFA also draws from the concepts and principles of numerous sciences and disciplines, including police and military science, criminal justice, criminology, sociology, human psychology, philosophy, histrionics, kinesics, proxemics, kinesiology, emergency medicine, crisis management, and human anatomy.

Sammy Franco has frequently been featured in martial art magazines, newspapers, and appeared on numerous radio and television programs. Mr. Franco has also authored numerous books, magazine articles and editorials, and has developed a popular library of instructional videos.

Sammy Franco's experience and credibility in the combat science is unequaled. One of his many accomplishments in this field includes the fact that he has earned the ranking of a Law Enforcement Master Instructor, and has designed, implemented, and taught officer survival training to the United States Border Patrol (USBP). He instructs members of the US Secret Service, Military Special Forces, Washington DC Police Department, Montgomery County, Maryland Deputy Sheriffs, and the US Library of Congress Police. Sammy Franco is also a member of the prestigious International Law Enforcement Educators and Trainers Association (ILEETA) as well as the American Society of Law Enforcement Trainers (ASLET) and he is listed in the "Who's Who Director of Law Enforcement Instructors."

Sammy Franco is a nationally certified Law Enforcement Instructor in the following curricula: PR-24 Side-Handle Baton, Police Arrest and Control Procedures, Police Personal Weapons Tactics, Police Power Handcuffing Methods, Police Oleoresin Capsicum Aerosol Training (OCAT), Police Weapon Retention and Disarming Methods, Police Edged Weapon Countermeasures and "Use of Force" Assessment and Response Methods.

Mr. Franco is also a National Rifle Association (NRA) instructor who specializes in firearm safety, personal protection and advanced combat pistol shooting.

Mr. Franco holds a Bachelor of Arts degree in Criminal Justice from the University of Maryland. He is a regularly featured speaker at a number of professional conferences, and conducts dynamic and enlightening seminars on numerous aspects of self-defense and personal protection.

For more information about Mr. Franco and his unique Contemporary Fighting Arts system, you can visit his website at: www.SammyFranco.com

If you liked this book, you will also want to read these:

FIRST STRIKE
End a Fight in Ten Seconds or Less!
by Sammy Franco

Learn how to stop any attack before it starts by mastering the art of the preemptive strike. First Strike gives you an easy-to-learn yet highly effective self-defense game plan for handling violent close-quarter combat encounters. First Strike will teach you instinctive, practical and realistic self-defense techniques that will drop any criminal attacker to the floor with one punishing blow. By reading this book and by practicing, you will learn the hard-hitting skills necessary to execute a punishing first strike and ultimately prevail in a self-defense situation. And that's what it is all about: winning in as little time as possible. 8.5 x 5.5, paperback, photos, illustrations, 202 pages.

OUT OF THE CAGE
A Complete Guide to Beating a Mixed Martial Artist on the Street
by Sammy Franco

Forget the UFC! The truth is, a street fight is the "ultimate no holds barred fight" often with deadly consequences, but you don't need to join a mixed martial arts school or become a cage fighter to defeat a mixed martial artist on the street. What you need are solid skills and combat proven techniques that can be applied under the stress of real world combat conditions. Out of the Cage takes you inside the mind of the MMA fighter and reveals all of his weaknesses, allowing you to quickly exploit them to your advantage. 10 x 7, paperback, photos, illustrations, 194 pages.

KUBOTAN POWER
Quick and Simple Steps to Mastering the Kubotan Keychain
by Sammy Franco

In this unique book, world-renowned self-defense expert, Sammy Franco takes thirty years of real-world teaching experience and gives you quick, easy and practical kubotan techniques that can be used by civilians, law enforcement personnel, or military professionals. Kubotan Power teaches you: tactical flashlight conversions, combat applications, grips, essential do's and don'ts, weapon nomenclature, impact shock, self-defense stages, high and low concealment positions, weapon deployment, target awareness, vital targets and medical implications, use of force considerations, attributes of fighting, defensive techniques, takedowns, training and flow drills, ground fighting, and much more. Whether you are a beginner or advanced, student or instructor, Kubotan Power shows you how to protect yourself and your loved ones against any thug you're likely to encounter on the street. 8.5 x 5.5, paperback, photos, illustrations, 204 pages.

WAR MACHINE
How to Transform Yourself Into A Vicious & Deadly Street Fighter
by Sammy Franco

War Machine is a book that will change you for the rest of your life! When followed accordingly, War Machine will forge your mind, body and spirit into iron. Once armed with the mental and physical attributes of the War Machine, you will become a strong and confident warrior that can handle just about anything that life may throw your way. In essence, War Machine is a way of life. Powerful, intense, and hard. 11 x 8.5, paperback, photos, illustrations, 210 pages.

THE COMPLETE BODY OPPONENT BAG BOOK
by Sammy Franco

In this one-of-a-kind book, world-renowned martial arts expert, Sammy Franco teaches you the many hidden training features of the body opponent bag that will improve your fighting skills and accelerate your fitness and conditioning. Develop explosive speed and power, improve your endurance, and tone, and strengthen your entire body. With detailed photographs, step-by-step instructions, and dozens of unique workout routines, The Complete Body Opponent Bag Book is the authoritative resource for mastering this lifelike punching bag. 8.5 x 5.5, paperback, photos, illustrations, 206 pages.

WHEN SECONDS COUNT
Self-Defense for the Real World
by Sammy Franco

When Seconds Count is a comprehensive street smart self-defense book instructing law abiding citizens how to protect themselves against the mounting threat of violent crime. When Seconds Count is considered by many to be one of the best books on real world self-defense instruction. Ideal for men and women of all ages who are serious about taking responsibility for their own safety. By studying the concepts and techniques taught in this book, you will feel a renewed sense of empowerment, enabling you to live your life with greater confidence and personal freedom. 10 x 7, paperback, photos, illustrations, 208 pages.

CONTEMPORARY FIGHTING ARTS, LLC
"Real World Self-Defense Since 1989"
www.SammyFranco.com
301-279-2244

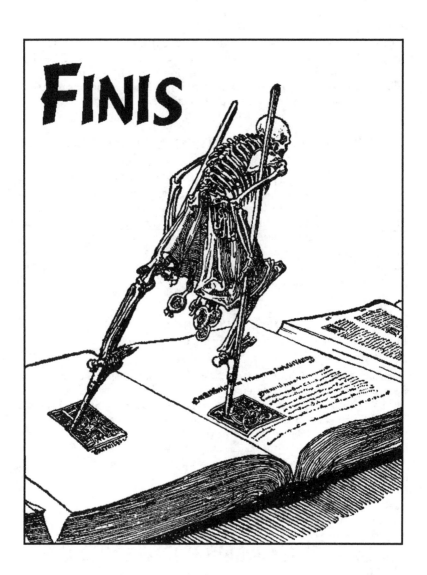